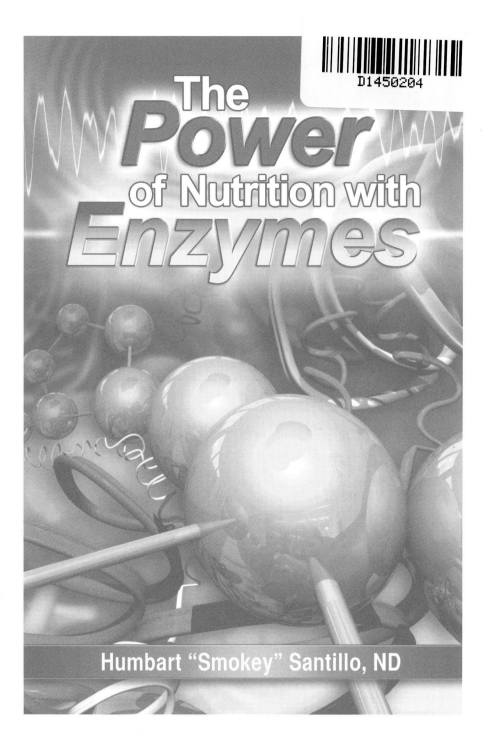

The
Power
of Nutrition with
Enzymes

D1450204

Humbart "Smokey" Santillo, ND

Designs for Wellness Press
Carlsbad, California © 2010

First Edition
Copyright © April 2010
by Humbart Santillo, N.D.

ISBN: 978-0-9641952-8-8

Designs for Wellness Press
P.O. Box 1671
Carlsbad, CA 92018-1671
888-796-5229

Editors: Kate B. Johnson, B.A., and Roy E. Vartabedian, Dr.P.H.

The information in this book reflects the author's experience and current research. It is not intended to be used to replace or supersede individualized medical or professional advice. Before starting any new nutrition or health program, you should consult a physician or other appropriate health professional to supervise your overall medical program.

Cover Illustration and Design by Eric Lindley
www.PartnersPhoto.com

Index by Madge Walls
www.AllSkyIndexing.com

Printed in the United States of America

Other publications by Dr. Santillo:

Herbal Combinations from Authoritative Sources
Natural Healing with Herbs
Natural Healing Herbal Correspondence Course
Intuitive Eating: Everybody's Guide to Lifelong Health and Vitality Through Food
The Basics of Intuitive Eating
Food Enzymes: The Missing Link to Radiant Health
ProMetabolics: Your Personal Guide to Transformational Health and Healing
Your Body Speaks—Your Body Heals

Visit Dr. Santillo's Web site: **www.SmokeySantillo.com   888-796-5229**
Volume discounts available.

DEDICATION

To Tony Collier,
National Enzyme Company
(Forsythe, MO)

When a man needs answers, he must reach out
and seek from those who are closest to him.
This man provided me with this blessing for years.
Thanks, my friend.

TABLE OF CONTENTS

FOREWORD

As one of the world's leading authorities on food enzymes, Dr. Smokey Santillo is uniquely qualified to write and teach about this highly important topic. In working with more than 30,000 patients as a naturopathic physician, he has witnessed first-hand the benefits of food enzymes, and the many maladies that occur in their absence.

We've all heard about vitamins and minerals, even phytochemicals—but we don't hear about enzymes much in the media. Dr. Santillo highlights the critical importance of these natural keys to unlocking energy and vitality for all people in modern society.

In *The Power of Nutrition with Enzymes*, he explains everything from the functions of enzymes to their myriad benefits for optimal health and longevity. This is the most accurate, comprehensive guide available for the layperson and an excellent, practical guide for professionals. Dr. Santillo has scoured the literature to bring you the important, useful information: how to preserve your body's natural enzyme stores, how to get enzymes from the right foods, and how you'll benefit from adding them to your diet.

If you want everything working for you as a peak-functioning human machine—leading a long, active, disease-free life—follow Dr. Santillo's advice. That's him on the back cover in track competition, a vibrant man and still a Masters world-class sprinter today. He practices what he preaches—and now you know his edge. I urge you to grab it for yourself.

Roy E. Vartabedian, Dr.P.H, M.P.H.
Doctor of Public Health, Preventive Care
President, Designs for Wellness

Author of New York Times Bestseller
Nutripoints: Healthy Eating Made Simple!
www.Nutripoints.com

INTRODUCTION:
THE POWER OF NUTRITION WITH ENZYMES

Throughout my years of experience as a health practitioner, author, and researcher, I developed a certain understanding: no singular formula, food, or health product is a "cure-all." And yet, though I intellectually knew this to be true, I still firmly believed there must be something that everyone could use as a health supplement, which could act as a nutritional foundation and even as an adjunct to medical and nonmedical therapies. Now I feel that my wish has come true. I found that what I was searching for was food enzymes.

Dr. Viktoras Kulvinskas, author of *Survival Into the 21st Century*,[21] sent me a book written by Dr. Edward Howell, *Food Enzymes for Health and Longevity*.[11] Dr. Howell's book explained to me why some therapies work and why some don't—because of enzymes. Enzymes are needed for every chemical action and reaction in the body. Enzymes are a part of all metabolic processes, from the working of our cells, tissues, and organs to the functioning of our digestive system, endocrine system, immune system, and every other system. Even minerals, vitamins, hormones, and neurotransmitters need enzymes to be present in order to do their own work properly. Enzymes are the true labor force of the body.

If you're interested in longevity, vitality, superior health, losing weight, or overcoming sickness—or if you feel that after taking vitamins and minerals for years, you haven't really benefited as much as you'd like to—this book is for you. The human machine has an innumerable amount of enzymes, and we will be hearing more and more about them. As we grow more health-conscious, we will certainly strive for a greater enjoyment of life. More energy and a stronger mind and body are needed to face the stresses the future will bring. Enzymes can be instrumental in achieving these goals. You'll be amazed by what these little creations of nature can do!

"The best consumer is an educated consumer..." We've all heard statements like this. The more educated we become about our health and how to take care of ourselves, the more guaranteed our future health will be. After all, your health is your responsibility. Keep educating your-self—it's a non-stop process. Love your body, respect it, help others to do the same, and stay well.

ENZYME BASICS: WHAT, HOW, WHERE, AND WHEN

In 1966, this statement appeared in a Scottish medical journal: "Each of us, as with all living organisms, could be regarded as an orderly, integrated succession of enzyme reactions."[11] We usually think of enzymes—if we think of them at all—as involved in digestion. And indeed, they are essential in digesting food and releasing nutrients to the body. But very seldom are we reminded that enzymes are also involved in every other metabolic function.

Enzymes are present throughout our tissues and organs. Our immune system, bloodstream, liver, kidneys, spleen, and pancreas, our ability to see, think, and breathe—all of our systems depend on enzymes. Nothing in the body can happen without them.

An enzyme shortage is very detrimental and may cause serious health problems. In fact, enzyme depletion can be as predisposing to disease as genetics or toxicity. Furthermore, as we become enzyme-deficient, we age faster. The more we build up our body's enzyme reserve, the healthier we'll be!

What Is an Enzyme? What Is Enzyme Activity?

In a nutshell, enzymes are energetic protein molecules. To describe their properties, I'll start with an analogy: A light bulb can only light up when an electric current flows through it. It is animated by electricity—the current is the "life force" of the bulb. Without electricity, it's just an object, without light. So a light bulb has a dual nature: a physical structure, and a nonphysical force that manifests itself through that structure.

The same idea applies to enzymes. An enzyme is a protein molecule, but that's not all; it has an activity. Each enzyme acts a certain way and does a certain job, whether that's digesting starch, building bones or skin, or aiding detoxification (to name only a few enzyme activities). When exposed to a high temperature, however, an enzyme is destroyed or denatured—that is, altered in such a way that it no longer carries out its designated function. Although the physical molecule is still present, it has lost its life force.

This "animated" property of enzymes was first observed in 1933, in chemistry experiments showing that the invisible "energy factor" of one protein molecule was transferred to another, leaving the original devoid of its former activity.[39] So for clarity, let's say that an enzyme's protein molecule is the "carrier" for the enzyme's activity, much like a light bulb is a carrier for electricity.

An enzyme acts upon a substance and changes it into another substance or a by-product, but the enzyme's identity remains unchanged. Any substance that an enzyme acts upon is called a substrate. Each enzyme is thought to fit geometrically with its corresponding substrate, as shown in Diagram 1.

How an Enzyme Works

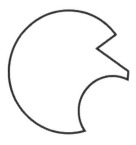

Enzyme Before Working

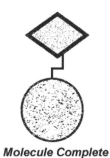

Molecule Complete

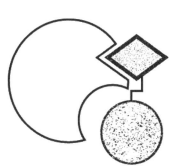

Enzyme While Working

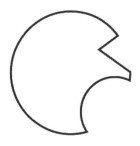

Enzyme After Working

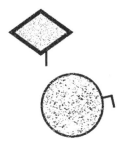

Molecule Split Apart

Diagram 1

Numbers and Names

For our purposes, the three major classes of enzymes are:

- metabolic enzymes (working in the body's blood, tissues, and organs)
- digestive enzymes (produced in the body for digestion)
- food enzymes (contained in raw food)

Since 1968, more than 1,300 enzymes have been identified. One researcher found 98 enzymes working in the arteries alone. To classify the burgeoning number of enzymes, the National Enzyme Commission devised a system of nomenclature, in which the name usually reveals the function and ends in the syllable "ase." Thus, the four categories of digestive enzymes are:[11]

- amylase—acts on starch (polysaccharides such as amylose and amylopectin)
- cellulase—acts on cellulose (plant fiber)
- lipase—acts on fat (lipids)
- protease— acts on protein

Each category includes a number of specific enzymes. For example, trypsin and pepsin, which act on proteins, are in the protease category. (Those two were identified before the nomenclature was implemented; to conform to that naming system, they're sometimes called trypsinogenase and pepsinogenase.) Proteases are also called proteolytic enzymes.

Don't get bogged down in the verbiage—remembering all the numbers and names is not important. What's important is understanding their sources, understanding how to get them into your body, and understanding that without them, life cannot exist.

What Do Enzymes Do in the Body?

Enzymes do a tremendous amount of work. In addition to breaking down foods and building the digested nutrients into healthy tissue, enzymes have numerous other duties. They are involved in every bodily process, and life could not exist without them. All cellular activity is initiated by enzymes. Here are a few examples that exemplify their importance to our everyday functions:[10]

- Enzymes assist in storing sugar as glycogen in the liver and muscles, and storing lipids in fatty tissue.
- One enzyme incorporates phosphorus into bone and nerve tissue; another helps to attach iron to red blood cells.
- Enzymes aid in the metabolism of nitrogen compounds into urea for excretion through urine, and also help to throw off carbon dioxide through the lungs.
- Enzymes in the immune system attack and eliminate wastes, poisons, and invaders in the blood and tissues.
- Sperm gain entrance to an ovum by carrying enzymes that dissolve tiny crevices in the ovum's membrane.

The sheer number of different enzymes in the body is overwhelming, yet each has a particular function. Enzymes are very "intelligent" when it comes to their activity. A protein-digestive enzyme will not digest a fat; a fat-digestive enzyme will not digest a starch. This is called enzyme specificity.

Where Do We Get Our Enzymes?

Enzymes are a component of all living matter and are integral to plant and animal life. Our endogenous metabolic and digestive enzymes are produced within the body by various organs and tissues. For example, the pancreas, which is of primary importance to the digestive system, secretes lipase, amylase, and protease to break down fat, starch, and protein.

The question is: Does the pancreas produce all of these enzymes itself? Logic dictates that an organ weighing only a few ounces (the average pancreas weighs only 85 grams) could not possibly be responsible for producing the enormous amount of enzymes needed by a 150-pound man day after day, year after year.

Early experiments showed that even when the pancreas is removed, the body still maintains a certain enzyme level. At the University of Toronto, a group of dogs were kept alive by the use of insulin after pancreas removal, and were shown to have normal blood levels of amylase.[11] At the Yale School of Medicine, dogs with their pancreatic ducts ligated (tied off) actually showed a rise in blood amylase of 20 times the normal amount.[15] The enzyme levels maintained in the absence of pancreatic contribution must come from somewhere else.

It has been substantiated that the pancreas receives enzymes from the blood and other tissues. Dr. Richard Willstatter demonstrated that leukocytes—white blood cells, which travel throughout the body as part of the immune system, destroying foreign substances—have amylase and proteolytic enzymes similar to those of the pancreas.[40] In fact, leukocytes contain an even greater variety of enzymes than the pancreas.

We inherited an enzyme reserve at birth and continue to produce enzymes through life, but this quantity can be decreased as we age, especially by eating an enzyme-deficient diet. If most of the food we eat is cooked, our system has to produce all of the enzymes needed for digestion. To supply them, the digestive organs must draw on the body's enzyme reserve in all organs and tissues, causing a deficit of metabolic enzymes.

Fortunately, nature has placed enzymes in food to aid in the digestive process instead of forcing our bodies to do all the work. We ingest exogenous enzymes from raw foods and as supplements derived from plant, animal, and fungal sources. Animals in the wild consume large amounts of enzymes in their primarily raw-food diets, taking unwarranted stress off their organs, which would otherwise decrease their longevity.

Enzymes Are Absorbed from the Intestines into the Bloodstream

A point of paramount importance is that a percentage of any enzymes eaten in raw food or taken orally as a supplement can be absorbed through the intestinal wall into the bloodstream and utilized (or stored) by the body, thereby helping to prevent enzyme depletion and taking stress off the enzyme-producing organs.

Dr. Anton W. Oelgoetz and colleagues found that when patients with low blood amylase were given an amylase-containing pancreatic extract, the normal blood amylase level was restored within 1 hour and remained normal for days after administration. Furthermore, when pancreatic enzymes were given to patients who had allergies and low blood enzyme levels, these levels returned to normal and the allergies subsided.[26]

Digestive disturbances, hyperacidity, and skin diseases caused by incompletely digested food materials can be effectively relieved the same way. The bloodstream provides an ideal environment for enzymes to break down undigested materials. Orally administered proteolytic enzymes have been used for years by Drs. Max Wolf and Karl Ransberger in treating inflammation and sports injuries.

Their book *Enzyme Therapy*[41] describes an experiment in which certain enzymes were tagged with radioactive dye to be followed through the digestive tract into the bloodstream and body. This electrophoretic investigation showed that the ingested enzymes turned up in the liver, spleen, kidneys, heart, lungs, and small intestine.

Where Do Enzyme Deficiencies Start?

One characteristic of enzymes is an inability to withstand hot temperatures, such as those in cooking. When live food substances contact heated water, their enzymes are denatured or destroyed quite rapidly. At 129°F, all enzymes are destroyed—that means there is no enzymatic activity in all foods that are canned, pasteurized, boiled, baked, roasted, stewed, or fried. Canned foods may still contain vitamins and minerals, but the heating process has killed the enzymes.

According to Dr. Howell, "Enzymes are more or less completely destroyed when heated in water in the temperature range between 48° to 65°C. Long heating at 48°C or short heating at 65°C kills enzymes. Heating at 60° to 80°C for one-half hour completely kills any enzymes."[11] Food processing, refining, cooking, and microwaving are detrimental processes that cause dramatic changes in the food we eat. They've rendered our foods enzyme-deficient, causing imbalances in our organs and acting as a predisposing cause of disease.

Investigations have shown that as temperature increases, enzymes work harder and are used up faster. For example, when starch-digesting enzymes are added to potato starch at a temperature of 80°F, the starch is digested much more rapidly than at a temperature of 40°F.[11]

The prevalent thought now is that enzymes are not actually "used up," but they are "lost" nonetheless. For example, many tests have shown that various enzymes are found in the urine after the heat of fevers and athletic activity. We lose enzymes every day through our sweat, urine, feces, and all digestive fluids, including salivary and intestinal secretions. And unfortunately, our body's enzyme reserve typically declines with age.

Other food substances, such as vitamins and minerals, are often replaced through our daily food intake, but not enough attention is placed on taking enzyme supplements or eating raw food. If we do not replenish our enzyme level from without, we defeat ourselves, as the body must then take enzymes from within itself—which in the end causes exhaustion, premature aging, and a low-energy system.

Depleted Soil, Depleted Food

Enzymes are present in the soil—amylase, lipase, urease, protease, cellulase, and more along—with bacteria and other microorganisms to continue supplying them. Earthworms make a huge enzyme contribution as they burrow, engulf soil's usable material, and excrete enzyme-rich "castings." Horticulturists look for soils with plentiful worm castings to cultivate their plants. Scientists measure enzymes in the soil to determine its health, which has a direct relationship to human nutrition.

For eons, countless animals replenished the Earth with enzyme-rich urine and feces. When the animals died, their rotting bodies supplied more enzymes to the soil. Before synthetic fertilizers were developed about 60 years ago, farmers used enzyme-rich manure. Organic farms are working hard to bring back this natural cycle.

Normally in nature, predators would remove the weakest members of the animal and plant kingdoms. The strongest animals and plants would survive, and they would be the healthiest—high in vitality and good nutrition for us. But in modern agriculture, this law of natural selection is now overridden, as farmers use powerful poisons to kill the predators, sparing the weak. Crops would not survive at all today if not for pesticides. In other words, modern plants, our fruits and vegetables, can no longer "stand on their own two feet."

Just think: we eat these weak plants, low in enzymes, low in energy, and even partly in a diseased state, and our livestock eat these plants too. The weaknesses are transferred to us. Our immune systems are weakening, and we now cannot live on food alone. Supplements and drugs are almost a necessity. Look at how many epidemics we have today—from heart disease, cancer, and circulatory problems, to the cluster of pancreatic diseases called Syndrome X. Overcooked foods, fast foods, enzyme-less plants, and chemicals have weakened our bodies to the point that we're all taking something to survive. It's no longer survival of the fittest; it's more like who's going to live the longest synthetically.

How Do We Counteract Enzyme Deficiency?

It is critical to preserve and replenish the body's enzyme level. There are two ways to do this: eating raw and predigested food, and taking supplemental enzymes. The tremendous value of these foods and supplements is discussed throughout this book. We must first try our best to get the most of the natural enzymes in foods by eating more raw, organically grown foods, and by avoiding fast foods and other processed foods.

But even with our best efforts, dietary improvement may not be enough. We need enzymes from outside sources. If we take in more exogenous enzymes, our enzyme reserve will not be depleted at such a rapid pace, and our body's metabolic enzymes will remain more evenly distributed. This is one of the most health-promoting measures that we can implement in our daily lifestyle.

My opinion is that anybody who eats cooked food should take digestive enzymes. If you're trying to build up your enzyme level to improve digestion, take them immediately before meals, and check the label to be sure the formula combines the whole family of digestive enzymes. (This is why I added amylase, protease, lipase, and cellulase to Juice Plus+®.)

ENZYMES AND DIGESTION

The thermodynamics of food concern energy in the form of biochemical compounds. The original source of that energy is the sun, as its electromagnetic energy is trapped in natural chemicals during photosynthesis. Humans, like all animals, can break down foods to release this energy at the cellular level, and use it to drive the energy-requiring processes of life. We are maintained not by the food we eat but by the food we actually digest. Food must be broken down by enzymes into simpler building blocks, or it is useless.

The energy in foods is our main energy source. We may think we're eating good foods, because they contain all the right vitamins and minerals, but we fail to consider whether the food's life force is still present. Its energy can be destroyed by cooking and processing. Over time, consuming such food has deleterious effects and even leads to illnesses, such as diabetes, cancer, and heart disease.

One of our main priorities in living a healthy life is to sustain our energy and prevent the exhaustion of our life force. This can be done by eating raw and predigested foods that bring sun-trapped vitality into our bodies. When we eat these foods, more nutrients and energy are available to us. Plus, the more exogenous enzymes we get, the less energy and endogenous enzymes we need to synthesize or borrow from other organs and metabolic processes.

Digestive Benefits of Raw Food

The difference between live (raw) and dead food is enzymatic activity. If you had two seeds and boiled one, which seed would grow when placed in soil? There is no question that the unboiled seed would sprout, because its enzymes are still intact.

All foods provided by nature have an abundance of enzymes when in their raw state. These enzymes contained in raw food are released through chewing and actually aid in the digestion of that same food. The enzymes inherent in raw food digest 5–75 percent of it themselves, without the help of enzymes secreted by the body. For instance, although fowl do not have amylase (starch-digestive enzyme), a study at the Agriculture College in Berlin fed chickens ground raw barley, which is very starchy, and analysis of the stomach contents after 5 hours showed that 8 percent of the starch was nevertheless digested.[10]

Because the enzymes contained in raw food help to digest it and can also be absorbed from the digestive tract into the bloodstream for use in other metabolic processes, we can conclude that taking supplemental enzymes and/or eating a large percentage of raw food will take significant stress off not only the pancreas, but the entire system. This is an example of energy conservation.

Another point is that compared to eating cooked food, less stomach acid is secreted when raw food is eaten. This allows the food enzymes to function optimally, with more time for predigestion. But when food is cooked and its enzymes destroyed, the food substrate remains inactive in the predigestive portion of the stomach. And if it is fatty or starchy, it must wait to pass into the small intestine before most of it is digested. When digestion is sluggish or enzyme levels are low (as often occurs in elderly folks), food ferments in the body, causing gas, bloating, constipation, colitis, and other problems.

These facts indicate that a vegetarian diet with at least 75 percent raw food is favorable. If this amount of raw food cannot be tolerated, plant-derived enzyme supplements can be used. Even eating an all raw-food diet may not guarantee enough enzymes, because citrus fruits and non-starchy vegetables contain small amounts of enzymes compared to starchy bananas, mangos, and avocados. So the raw-foodist can benefit from taking plant enzymes as well. Knowing how to use raw foods and supplemental enzymes is a tremendous dietary advantage. (For information on the healing effects of raw foods, see the works of well-known naturalists Arnold Ehret, Ann Wigmore, George Drews, and Viktoras Kulvinskas.)

What Is Digested Where, and Why?

Popular opinion formerly held that the acid in the stomach destroyed any enzymes eaten in food or taken as oral supplements, and that the only nutritional value of ingested enzymes is their constituent amino acids. This is simply not true.[39] Research has proven that some ingested enzymes are active in the stomach, some in the intestine, and some in both. Amylase, for example, functions throughout the digestive tract; a study at Northwestern University showed that a barley-derived amylase supplement digested starch in the stomach, then passed unharmed into the small intestine, where it continued digestion.[5] Dr. Ismar Boas demonstrated that "the enzymes in bananas were activated in the intestines to aid in the digestive process."[10] A Russian researcher, Dr. Matveev, similarly demonstrated that the carrot enzymes oxidase and catalase were inactivated in the acidity of the stomach, and then reactivated in the alkalinity of the small intestines.[10]

Another longstanding misconception was that protein is the only food digested in the stomach, leaving fat and carbohydrate digestion to pancreatic secretions in the small intestine—but this has been disproven as well. In a study at the Illinois College of Medicine, Dr. Olaf Berglim gave human participants mashed potatoes and bread, which both contain large amounts of starch. When the stomach contents were retrieved after 45 minutes, 76 percent of the potato starch and 59 percent of the bread starch had been digested.[10] And research by Dr. J. M. Beazell and colleagues showed that several times more starch than protein was digested in the stomach within the first hour.[14]

The body's digestive organs and juices have characteristic pH ranges. What is pH? The acronym stands for "hydrogen potential." The more hydrogen is in a solution, the more acidic it is; and as hydrogen concentration decreases, a solution becomes more alkaline. So acid and alkaline describe ranges of pH. Numbers from 1 to 14 are used to denote degrees of acidity and alkalinity:

- 1–6 = acidic (1 is very acidic, 6 is slightly acidic)
- 7 = neutral
- 8–14 = alkaline (8 is slightly alkaline, 14 is very alkaline)

The stomach's digestive juices include hydrochloric acid (HCl) and have an overall pH range of 1.6–4.0. Dr. W. H. Taylor of Oxford University discovered two distinct pH zones in the stomach. In the first, "predigestive" region of the stomach, the pH range is mildly acidic, at 3.4–4.0. Lower in the stomach, the pH becomes more acidic, ranging approximately 1.6–2.4.[36]

Dr. Taylor also found that the body's pepsin (a protease) functions best in a pH range of 1.5–2.5. This means that at the beginning of digestion, pepsin is not at optimum capability and has little activity. As food moves into the more acidic region of the stomach, approximately 1/2–1 hour after being eaten, pepsin's digestive activity increases. As it turns out, the body begins to digest protein in the stomach, and then continues the process in the small intestine.

Once the food in the stomach becomes a semi-fluid paste called chyme, it passes slowly into the small intestine. In the first part of that organ, called the duodenum, pancreatic secretions containing bicarbonate ions neutralize the pepsin and the chyme's initial acidity, and change the pH to a more alkaline range, around 7–8. Pancreatic and intestinal enzymes function best in an alkaline environment.

At this point, trypsin, a pancreatic enzyme that also digests protein, is secreted into the small intestine and basically takes over where pepsin leaves off. The pancreas also secretes amylase and lipase into the small intestine to digest fats and carbohydrates.

Animal-, Plant-, and Fungus-Derived Enzyme Supplements

Of the many enzyme supplements on the market, some are better than others. Finding the most suitable supplements to substitute for deficient endogenous enzymes is of primary importance. Given that most digestion occurs in the stomach and small intestine, enzymes with activity in a wider pH range are much more beneficial than those active in only one organ. Enzymes are needed that can work in the predigestive stomach, lower stomach, and small intestine.

Diagram 2 illustrates the pH ranges in which various types of digestive enzymes function best:

EFFECTIVE pH RANGES

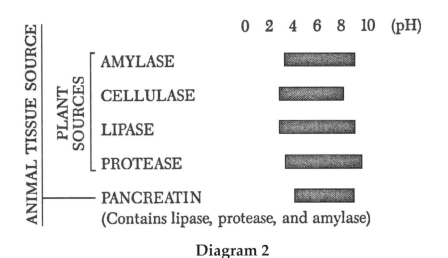

Diagram 2

"Pancreatin" is a collective term for pancreatic secretions containing lipase, protease, and amylase combined. Pancreatin supplements are usually extracted, purified, and concentrated from slaughterhouse animals. As you can see, animal-derived pancreatin cannot function in a wide range of pH. It can only function in the alkaline small intestine, not the more acidic stomach.

Supplemental pancreatin is usually contained in enteric-coated capsules, which are treated in such a way as to pass through the stomach's acidity inactive and unchanged—without participating in stomach digestion. Not until the intestine do alkaline juices dissolve the coating and release the enzymes. Because this release is triggered by pancreatic secretion, supplemental pancreatin does not take stress off the pancreas as much as plant-derived enzymes do.

It was formerly postulated that enzymes extracted from plants could not substitute for tissue-derived enzyme extracts, but scientists have proven otherwise. It has been established that certain plant-derived proteases and lipases can function in a wide pH range of 3–8.5, predigesting a good percentage of the food in the stomach and then continuing digestion in the small intestine before the pancreas even secretes its enzymes. Thus, the pancreas has less work to do, and more enzymes can be preserved for other metabolic functions. This is a relief to the whole body. Plant-derived enzymes that digest protein, fat, and starch are available in most health food stores.

An interesting research paper compared bromelain, a proteolytic enzyme extracted from pineapples, to the body's own pepsin and trypsin.[9] Bromelain was found to have the same protein-digestive capabilities as pepsin and trypsin, and to be active not only in the stomach's pH range but also in the alkaline environment of the small intestine. Thus, bromelain can be effectively substituted for pepsin and trypsin in enzyme supplementation.

At the University of Texas, Dr. W. A. Selle studied a group of dogs with their pancreatic ducts ligated (tied off) so no pancreatic juices would affect digestion when they were then fed cereal starch with the addition of barley-derived amylase. In some cases, the cereal starch was 65 percent digested in the stomach. The barley-derived amylase digested starch in stomach pHs as acidic as 2.5; by comparison, salivary amylase could not function in an acidic pH as well as the barley amylase, being inactivated in the stomach at a pH of 4.5. And ½-hour after it was orally taken, 69–71 percent of the barley amylase was found in the small intestine, still actively digesting starch. Fecal matter was also found to contain more barley amylase than the dogs' own pancreatic enzymes.[10]

Enzymes from fungi (mushrooms and yeast) have been experimentally evaluated and shown to be very active in both the stomach and intestines, even the large intestine. Dr. Howell found that certain fungi, cultured on food materials such as wheat, bran, or soybeans, produce protease, lipase, amylase, and cellulase that can function in tremendously wide pH ranges. These fungal enzymes have been found to function throughout the intestinal tract, also helping to correct deficient blood enzyme patterns. Dr. Howell recommends chewing a few of these encapsulated enzymes with meals, or taking the powder in small amounts of water before eating.[11]

Deficits of Cooked and Overprocessed Food

A diet of mostly cooked food has proven to be detrimental in more ways than one. Cooking does not improve food's nutritional value—rather, it destroys or makes unavailable 85 percent of the food's original nutrients. Cooked food is totally lacking in enzymes; most of the protein has been destroyed, or converted to forms that are either not digestible by body enzymes or digested with difficulty; many of the vitamins have lost their vitality. To purchase organic food and then waste precious hours in destroying most of the nutrients is poor economy and unsound ecology.

Most food-processing techniques involve the application of heat—blanching, boiling, and irradiation (e.g., microwaving) are just a few. These processes not only remove the food's energy but also alter its important vitamins and minerals. Processing often destroys or denatures proteins, including enzyme proteins. Sometimes overheating causes a protein's amino acids to become cross-linked, and the body cannot recognize the altered protein as a food. If the body cannot use them or get rid of them, they're stored in the tissues and can cause future health problems.

The U.S. Department of Agriculture has a complete database on food thermodynamics before and after processing, and dramatic energy losses are observed. For example, 30 percent of the energy in green beans and carrots is lost during processing; meats and seafood can lose 7–31 percent; and dairy products can lose up to 50 percent.[41] Nutrient loss to cooking and processing is also tremendous. Grains can lose up to 15 percent of their protein, 65 percent of fat, 80 percent of thiamine, 40 percent of riboflavin, 66 percent of niacin, and 94 percent of vitamin B6.[41] Fruits can lose 40–70 percent of their vitamin C; peaches, for example, lose 70 percent of niacin, vitamin A and C, riboflavin, and thiamine. From blanching, spinach loses 35 percent of its water-soluble vitamins.[41]

Canning is most destructive. Comparative experiments at Columbia University showed that canned food, from being cooked and/or preserved, is completely devoid of enzymes.[18] Sometimes up to 90 percent of other specific nutrients are lost during this process as well.[18] I could go on all day on this subject; there's tons of research.

Consequences of a Cooked-Food Diet

Dr. Howell states, "Researchers show that cooked food with the fiber broken down passes through the digestive system more slowly than raw foods. Partially it ferments, rots, and putrefies, throwing back into the body toxins, gas, and causing heartburn and degenerative diseases."[10]

Cooked foods, especially those high in protein, can begin to putrefy. The byproducts of putrefaction are toxins, which are then absorbed into the bloodstream and eventually deposited at body sites far from the intestinal tract. At this point, you can see how valuable enzymes are in helping to keep the blood clear of poisons. It has been estimated that 80 percent of diseases are caused by the absorption of improperly digested foods and their by-products.[21]

Furthermore, if food is overcooked and its enzymes destroyed, the only enzymes that get mixed with the food in our predigestive stomach are the ones contained in saliva. Salivary amylase may enable some starch digestion. Although the food remains in the predigestive stomach for its allotted time, practically no other predigestion takes place. The protein is eventually acted upon by the stomach's pepsin, but as you now know, that occurs mostly in the lower part of the stomach. The fat remains practically untouched until it moves into the small intestine, where it encounters pancreatic lipase.

Cooked food exerts a powerful stimulating effect on the endocrine glands, leading them to become overworked and encouraging weight gain, hypoglycemia, and obesity. If the glands know the body has had enough calories, but the nutrients and enzymes that should accompany these calories aren't present because of food's overcooking, the glands respond to their absence with a disruptive endocrine imbalance. The glands also overstimulate the digestive organs, demanding more food than is actually needed to maintain the body's strength and vitality. The results are hormone oversecretion, overeating, obesity, and, finally, exhaustion of the glands and depletion of the enzyme reserve from carrying on all the increased metabolic activity.

Eating properly helps to counter unnecessary organ breakdown and malfunction, but you can see the overshadowing damage done by eating enzyme-free, overcooked food. Large amounts of enzymes are used up, leaving the organs and tissues without their rightful share. One can live for many years on a cooked-food diet, but eventually this causes cellular enzyme exhaustion, which lays the foundation for a weak immune system and, ultimately, disease. We all suffer the consequences of cooked-food diets—and so can other animals. Zoologists know that captured animals fed a cooked-food diet develop human diseases such as gastritis, duodenitis, colitis, liver disease, anemia, thyroid disease, arthritis, and circulatory problems.

Dr. Francis Pottenger carried out a ten-year experiment using 900 cats on controlled diets. The cats eating raw food produced healthy kittens from generation to generation. Those eating cooked food developed various ailments: heart, kidney, and thyroid disease, pneumonia, paralysis, loss of teeth, difficulty in labor, diminished or perverted sexual interest, diarrhea, and irritability. Liver impairment on cooked food was progressive, the bile becoming so toxic that even weeds couldn't grow in soil fertilized by the cats' excrement. The first generation was sickly and sluggish; the second generation developed degenerative diseases in midlife; many in the third generation were born dead or diseased, developed degenerative diseases that dramatically shortened their lives, or were sterile; and the fourth generation simply died out.[27]

Cooked Food and Pancreas Enlargement

It is interesting to observe that the pancreases of animals subsisting exclusively on raw plant material are much smaller (relative to body weight) than the human pancreas, as shown in Table 1.[11] The pancreas of a 140-pound human weighs 85–90 grams, whereas that of an 85-pound sheep weighs only 18.8 grams; that of a 1,005-pound cow, only 308 grams; and that of a 1,200-pound horse, only 330 grams.

	Body Weight (grams)	Pancreas Weight (% body weight)
Sheep	38,505	0.0490
Cow	455,265	0.0680
Horse	543,600	0.0603
Man	63,420	0.1400

Table 1

Notice how little a man's body weighs compared to a cow or horse, and yet how much larger his pancreas is. The human pancreas becomes enlarged when it is overworked by digesting a cooked-food diet devoid of enzymes. The fascinating point is that human saliva contains amylase to aid the pancreas in starch digestion, whereas herbivores have relatively no amylase in their saliva, and yet the animals' pancreases remain normal size. The reason seems to be that their raw food supplies active enzymes for digestion, thus taking stress off the pancreas, other digestive organs, and, in fact, the whole body's metabolism.

In 1933, 768 postmortem examinations at the Philippine School of Public Health found that the pancreases of the autopsied Filipinos were 25–50 percent heavier than those of the Europeans and Americans.[11] Cooked rice was their staple food, eaten as many as three times a day. This bulk overworked their pancreases, which became enlarged from secreting such great amounts of enzymes (particularly amylase). A cooked-food diet causes a larger outpouring of enzymes from our digestive organs. Though some might think hypertrophied (enlarged) organs are a desirable accommodation, it is often a pathological condition—an organ's enlargement is always accompanied by its excessive function, usually followed by its exhaustion and degeneration.

Cooked Food and Digestive Leukocytosis

Dr. Paul Kouchakoff, who studied the effect of cooking on our systems, found an increase in white blood cells after the ingestion of a cooked-food meal.[20] As all metabolic processes are interrelated at all times, this increased white blood cell count in response to cooked food—when the body must supply a large amount of digestive enzymes—indicates a compensatory measure to aid digestion. These extra leukocytes are needed to produce extra enzymes and transport them to the digestive tract.

Dr. Kouchakoff demonstrated that after a raw-food meal, there was no substantial leukocyte increase. Because enzymes in raw food help in digestion, the action of those enzymes removes the stress of having to borrow them from the body's reserve, particularly from the white blood cells, which are an important part of our immune systems. Leukocytosis, or increased white blood cell count, is an actual medical pathology. Whenever the white blood cell count increases to any great extent, an acute illness or infection is thought to be present somewhere in the body. It can also lead to weight gain. Clearly, in the long run, a cooked-food diet cannot be the best regimen to follow.

PREDIGESTION AND PREDIGESTED FOODS

If there's a missing link in the literature of nutrition, it is predigested food. Thousands of books and research papers claim that various herbs, foods, and supplements can be used for disease recovery, anti-aging, and immune system support. Predigested foods are not only represented in all of these nutritional categories but also constitute a category of "super-foods" all their own. If you're into nutrition at any level, you'll find this section to be one of the most exciting and informative you've ever read.

A predigested food is just what it sounds like—a food that's digested outside the body before it's eaten. This is a tremendous advantage, as it saves on the body's own digestive energy and resources. Naturally occurring predigested foods include sprouts and fruits—that is, their proteins, starches, and fats are already broken down before they're actually consumed. There are two major ways to make predigested foods: by fermentation, or by using enzymes.

Improving your diet by eating a good quantity of predigested foods can be hugely beneficial. When I talk about nutrition, I say that food has two levels of nutrition: an energetic level, and a physical substance level of carbohydrates, proteins, fats, vitamins, and minerals. Predigested foods supply both of these bodily needs. And in a predigested whole food, an entire orchestra of nutrients is available for the taking, in synergistic form. All vitamins and minerals need each other for bioavailability and for the body to function properly. I'm not saying, "Don't take individual vitamins and minerals"; I'm saying, "Do make sure your diet includes enough whole foods and predigested foods to compensate for any possible deficiency."

Very few foods are designed for everybody as pre-digested foods are. Whether you're an athlete, recovering from an illness, or simply interested in staying healthy and slowing the aging process, these foods will help you. Predigested foods have even been proven safe and health-promoting for infants. Possibilities for use include cereal, meal replacement, supplemental fiber, protein powder, hospital food, dietary aid for the elderly—the potential is endless.

The concept of predigestion has been around forever. It's one of those concepts that have always been the most obvious, yet we look the other way. It's too simple to be true, and too easy to understand. Something's got to be difficult to be worth it, or so we think—but not in this situation.

We're Designed for Predigestion

Nature has provided us with an anatomical structure and a physiology that naturally dictate eating predigested foods. The physiologist Walter B. Cannon demonstrated that the human stomach "consists of two parts physiologically distinct." He states: "The cardiac portion of the stomach is a food reservoir in which salivary digestion continues; the pyloric portion is the seat of active gastric digestion. There are no peristaltic waves in the cardiac portion."[4]

The upper portion of the stomach can be called the enzyme-stomach, and its importance cannot be over-estimated. In formal anatomical terms, our enzyme-stomach comprises the cardiac and fundic regions, illustrated in Diagram 3. No acid secretion or peristalsis takes place in the enzyme-stomach for ½–1 hour after food is eaten. This is when and where the natural enzymes contained in food, as well as any supplemental digestive enzymes, do their predigestive work.

Major Regions of the Stomach

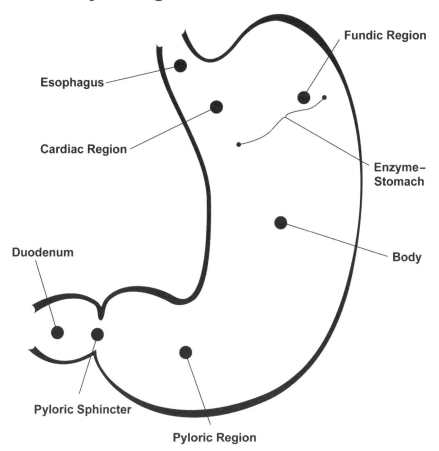

Diagram 3

Our enzyme potential has more useful (and taxing) work to do than making digestive enzymes to break down our food.[11] The more digestion is accomplished in the stomach, the less pancreatic and intestinal secretion is needed, thereby conserving our endogenous enzymes for other processes. The body is greatly relieved when predigestion takes place and the draw on metabolic enzymes is kept to a minimum.

Predigestion is widespread in nature, and the enzyme-stomach is not unique to humans. Of the four stomachs in cattle and sheep, only one secretes enzymes; the other three allow the enzymes in food to do the digesting. Dolphins and whales have three stomachs, including one devoid of its own enzymes. In one studied whale, as many as 32 seals were found in that enzyme-stomach—but with no enzyme secretion there, how could all that flesh be broken down enough to pass through a small opening to the other stomachs?

The answer is the enzymes in the flesh of the eaten animals. After death, animal tissues become acidic, causing the release of the enzyme cathepsin, which begins pre-digesting the proteins. Cathepsin and other enzymes are active for a long time. The animals that consume this predigested flesh benefit tremendously, as their own bodies don't have to secrete lots of enzymes to break down and utilize the food.

The Synergy of Exogenous and Endogenous Digestive Enzymes

A portion of the enzymes in raw foods survives passage into and through the human digestive tract, which means they can aid in predigestion. These enzymes can actually digest 5–75 percent of the food themselves. The enzymes in raw and predigested foodstuffs also work synergistically with those in the body to break down large molecules for absorption into the bloodstream and to release maximal energy from food.[10]

Research has shown that for the first 45 minutes to 1 hour, a good percentage of food can be predigested in the stomach before reaching the small intestine. At this time, the pancreas secretes protein-, fat-, and starch-digestive enzymes into the duodenum (the first part of the small intestine). If the food has not been properly predigested, the pancreas can be put under tremendous stress, as it must draw enzymes from throughout the body to secrete the amount needed for full digestion. The pancreas is one of the first organs to dysfunction in many chronic illnesses.

The more digestion takes place before food reaches the small intestine, the better for the integrity, strength, and immunity of the whole body. The body values its enzymes and will make no more than needed for the job. In accordance with the Law of Adaptive Secretion of Digestive Enzymes, the body can adjust the amount and type of enzymes it secretes according to the foods consumed. If the food's own enzymes are intact, or if the food is predigested before it's eaten, the body will secrete less.

The judicious distribution of enzyme energy helps to maintain health, slow aging, and prevent disease. Preserving the body's enzyme potential; making nutrients more available to the cells; making more enzymes available for metabolism, benefiting the endocrine and immune systems and improving cellular thermodynamics—all of this, accomplished simply by eating the foods we're naturally designed to consume!

The Tremendous Value and Many Uses of Predigested Food

Can you really eat enough raw food so the body doesn't have to use its enzyme reserves? That would be a lot of eating and a lot of food. A raw-food diet can be difficult to follow, especially as we age and don't have the digestive strength to break down hard, fibrous foods. Plus, replacing cooked foods with raw foods can seem like a lot of work. Many people also have blood types that demand the use of meats and heavier foods. Eating predigested food is a more efficacious way to prevent the body from depleting its enzymes.

All of our organs, tissues, and systems are largely dependent on our enzyme levels and affected by enzyme activity. Eating predigested food supports most bodily functions by not causing enzyme exhaustion. When the body doesn't have to work as hard in digestion, more energy is available for healing, stamina, and growth. For the enzymes lacking in our diet, predigested foods compensate a good percentage, helping to preserve our glandular system. That, in turn, affects aging, weight control issues, and much more. This anti-aging, anti-disease factor isn't much talked about in today's nutritional literature—but it's especially important, because as we get older, we become enzyme-deficient. Enzyme deficiencies are a bottom-line factor in most chronic disease, and many modern diseases are related to the pancreas.

Predigested food does not gelatinize, its granules are smaller, it's easier to digest, it yields more energy, and it leaves less food residue to eliminate. Its nutrient density is more than doubled as well.[11] Centuries of tradition in various cultures and no fewer than 60 research papers have verified the effects of these super-foods. Predigested foods are one of nature's greatest gifts, and give us a new way of looking at eating, health, and longevity.

Sometimes weight-loss diets don't work because their foods are enzyme-deficient, and because constantly eating small amounts of food can cause further enzyme depletion through continual digestive effort. Eating predigested foods, however, liberates more nutrients and enzymes to the body, resulting in less hunger, and the need for excessive eating can be diminished.

Athletes are now using predigested protein powders and predigested whole-food concentrates before and after their workouts, mainly because the nutrients are more bio-available (easier to absorb). Thus, the athlete has less food waste to eliminate, and has more energy available for faster recovery because less is used for digestion and cellular detoxification.

Don't you think predigested food should be used in hospitals for sick and recovering patients, so more body energy is available for healing instead of being used for digesting and eliminating waste from cooked and unnatural food? It's a "no-brainer" to use these foods during any sickness or chronic disease. They help to maintain health and stamina, support the immune system, and aid in recovery and muscle building. Very few food substances can match predigested foods for their versatility and compatibility in people from elders to infants. Infants and children can benefit from eating predigested foods in smoothies, fruit drinks, cereals, and meal replacements.

After reading this book, you'll understand the value of consuming predigested foods. These foods really can be classified as anti-aging substances! (For more information on raw-food diets, sprouting, and predigested foods, I recommend the works of Dr. Viktoras Kulvinskas, author of *Survival Into the 21st Century*.[21])

Predigested Foods Around the World

The predigestion concept is not new. Predigested foods have been used in many rural cultures for centuries and are still widely used today. In the absence of refrigeration, traditional cultures use fermentation and other techniques as a means of preserving the food supply and increasing its nutritional value. Fermented vegetables are enjoyed worldwide, from olives, pickled cucumbers, and sauerkraut, to Chinese *hum choy*, Japanese *zukemono*, and Korean *kim chi*, which has more than 50 varieties and goes back to the third century AD. Basically, raw vegetables such as cabbage and radishes are chopped up, mixed with spices, and allowed to ferment—so microorganisms and enzymes in the food eventually predigest it. Koreans consume about 90 grams per day of *kim chi* and use it to improve digestion and treat constipation; it is high in B vitamins and vitamin C, antimutagenic, and anticarcinogenic.

Asiatic peoples have also improved soybeans by predigesting them with fungal enzymes into foods such as *tempeh*, *tamari*, and *miso*. Cheeses and meats can be "aged" by enzymes too; in Lebanon, a dish of crushed raw lamb and wheat is set aside to predigest before it is eaten. Primitive Eskimos catch fish and bury it until it partially decays. The enzymes in the tissue predigest the fish, which is then unearthed and eaten. It's called "high fish" because it gives the Eskimos (and their dogs) strength and endurance. They don't have to secrete large amounts of enzymes to digest it, and the conservation of digestive energy leaves more for work, metabolic functions, thinking, and exercise.

Fermentation versus Enzymatic Predigestion

As mentioned, fermentation is a biochemical modification of primary food brought about by microorganisms and enzymes contained within the food. However, now that we strip our soils and foods of enzymes and use synthetic fertilizers, our deficient foods can greatly alter the fermentation process normally carried out by food's lactic-acid-producing bacteria.

Fermentation is also a risky way to predigest, as little quality control is possible when foods are fermented in the home. During fermentation, several acids and alcohols are produced (these don't develop during enzymatic pre-digestion), and, mycotoxins and endotoxins from certain bacteria and molds can also develop, especially when temperatures increase. In uncontrolled fermentation, these toxins and molds can produce untold chemical changes that can cause subclinical symptoms and initiate digestive problems.

I once visited a healing center where people were drinking fermented water drained off grains that had soaked for a short time. These people complained of nausea and stomach upset. The ferment showed high levels of unhealthy bacteria. Some acid-resistant bacteria can live through the fermentation process and produce other pathogens and contaminants.[39] It can be difficult to identify these microorganisms and contaminants until people get sick.

Enzymatic predigestion is by far the safer method and is a much more controlled process. Known enzymes from plant and animal sources are combined in a slurry with crushed, ground, or pulverized vegetables or grains and kept at a specific temperature for a specific length of time. After the enzymes break down the food, the temperature is increased for a few minutes, stopping the process. The resulting food is partially predigested and more bioavailable (absorbable). The nutrient content of some of these foods even increases.[11]

Using enzymes is more sophisticated but not always feasible. In rural areas, fermentation is mainly used, due to its simplicity and availability. Fermented cereals have long been used as weaning foods in African countries, including Nigeria, Kenya, and the United Republic of Tanzania.[11] Sorghum, millet, and maize are traditionally pounded, pulverized, and sieved into a flour-like substance, which is mixed with water and left in a vessel to ferment for 3–4 days. Other foods such as fish, meat, and vegetables are also predigested to add nutritional value to the diet. In a study of consumption of fermented foods among health workers and mothers of young children in rural and urban communities in Kenya, 83 percent in the rural areas reported regularly using these foods, compared to 56 percent in the urban areas.

Perhaps the most important property of fermented foods is their increased acidity, which is associated with reduced pathogens. African communities commonly use fermentation to reduce microbial contamination of porridges in an effort to prevent and manage diarrhea. Developing countries need a better weaning food to combat diarrhea and malnutrition, which are prevalent causes of childhood morbidity and mortality. In rural areas, diarrhea and dehydration cause 750,000 to 1 million deaths a year.

An experiment comparing the effectiveness of fermented and enzymatically predigested food was conducted with pediatric diarrhea at the Treatment Unit of the Muhimbili Medical Center in Tanzania.[11] Seventy-five children aged 6–25 months, admitted to the hospital with acute diarrhea, pneumonia, meningitis, septicemia, acute ear infection, and urinary tract infections, were split into three treatment groups. One group ate conventional sorghum porridge. The second group ate fermented sorghum porridge, and the third ate sorghum porridge predigested by amylase.

Evaluation of the energy intake from these foods showed that the first two groups had equal amounts of energy intake, whereas the group that ate the amylase-predigested porridge had 42 percent more, even though the children with the more severe illnesses were in this group. The amylase group was also able to tolerate their food better. Being able to consume more energy via predigested food is a hugely important issue in such cases.

Soaking and Sprouting:
The Only Way to Eat Seeds and Nuts

Soaking and sprouting grains, seeds, and nuts is another way to make predigested foods at home. (Check your health food store for books on sprouting.) The method seems easy, but it has pitfalls. It's time-consuming—not everybody can soak food 1–3 days and keep up with all the sprouting for a whole family—and you'll need to be creative so the foods won't become boring. More importantly, acids and contaminants are produced in soaking, and mold can develop. Only organic foods should be used, and the environment should be kept absolutely sterile. If you're sick or fatigued, this can be a lot of work.

Seeds, nuts, and grains contain enzymes, proteins, fats, hormone precursors, and minerals. But they also contain enzyme inhibitors, chemical compounds which are released during the predigestion process (soaking and sprouting). If the process is not done correctly, the inhibitors can remain in the food (or in the soaking solution) and interfere with subsequent breakdown of its protein and starch.

Because enzymes are very active entities, nature has to put a rein on them in seeds until the necessary environment for germination and plant growth is provided. Inhibitors keep enzymes dormant until the seed is adequately moistened and buried in soil. When that happens, the inhibitors are released, freeing the enzymes from bondage, so they can digest the seed's fats, carbohydrates, and proteins to feed the eventual sprout. Here is nature's inherent predigestive plan: a seed high in protein has protein inhibitors; a seed high in starch has starch inhibitors; a seed high in fat has fat inhibitors; and seeds high in all three have all three types of inhibitors.

The mistake we make is eating seeds and nuts before their inhibitors are released or neutralized. To compensate for the inhibitors, the pancreas must secrete an over-abundance of digestive enzymes. This causes enzyme exhaustion throughout the body, depleting the blood and endocrine system of enzymes. Experiments have shown that when inhibitors are eaten, enzymes are wasted by excretion through the feces. It's a double-edged sword. The body cannot use the enzymes in the food, and the pancreas gets depleted and overworked. At the University of California at Berkeley, researchers Samuel Lepkovsky and Fred Furuta demonstrated this in an experiment feeding chickens raw soybeans containing enzyme inhibitors; the birds failed to grow or gain body weight, and yet their pancreases became more than twice as heavy as normal, and their enzyme output markedly increased.[23]

This is also what happens when enzyme inhibitors called starch blockers are used to prevent the body's assimilation of starch. Ingesting any type of enzyme inhibitor results in a huge withdrawal from the enzyme "bank account," and interfering with the normal function of the body in this way is never a good idea. That's what's wrong with a lot of the cereals and meal-replacement products on the market. Processing doesn't always neutralize the inhibitors, and heating the seeds, nuts, or grains destroys all the enzymes. Surely nutrient-deficient foods loaded with inhibitors are not anti-aging or healthful!

Experimental Evidence of Grain Predigestion

The human digestive tract has evolved complicated but efficient mechanisms to digest and release maximum energy from a wide variety of foodstuffs. An excellent model system has been developed to understand this complex process by measuring the nutritional value of foodstuffs prior to eating and then following their digestion through the small intestine. This can be done with patients who have had an ileostomy (surgical removal of the large intestine), as the contents of the small intestine can be analyzed to discern the digestive efficiency of any diet. Significant support for the enzyme-synergy theory has been gained from these patients.

Whole grains and cereals are difficult to digest because they contain phytate, a non-nutrient component of plants, seeds, grains, and the husks of grains and legumes. In the body, phytate binds with minerals such as zinc, iron, calcium, magnesium, and copper, leading to their excretion unused—which can lead to mineral deficiency. Fortunately, the enzyme phytase, which occurs naturally in these foods, breaks down phytate.

Heating grain to 120°C, however, destroys its endogenous phytase. Analysis revealed that 95 percent of the phytate was retained in the ileostomy contents when a group of these patients ate heated grain, whereas only 40 percent of the phytate remained from eating unheated grain.[10] This shows that endogenous phytase is necessary for proper digestion and release of energy from grain.

The same thing happens with all of our cooked foods as with those patients' heated grain—the enzymes (and other nutrients) are destroyed, and the body struggles to survive. Don't you think this can have something to do with why so many of us experience fatigue and low energy?

Predigested Foods Improve the Body's Digestion of Protein and Fats

Predigested foods are not only partially digested themselves, but positively affect pancreatic secretion, intestinal pH, and release of the hormone cholecystokinin (CCK), which is secreted by the small intestine to stimulate pancreatic secretion and gallbladder contraction (aiding the digestion of fat). Imagine the health problems that ensue if these mechanisms fail us!

An experiment performed on a group of dogs investigated the effect of predigested food on pancreatic enzymes and CCK.[11] For 3 weeks, the dogs were fed cooked, strained liver, either partially predigested by added enzymes or non-predigested, and frequent samples of blood and duodenal fluid were taken. The results showed that eating predigested liver, compared to non-predigested liver, produced approximately three times the amount of pancreatic secretions containing bicarbonate and protein, as well as a significantly greater amount of pancreatic juice containing 20 times the amino acid content. Similarly, blood CCK concentration resulting from predigested liver was three times the amount resulting from non-predigested liver. This study clearly demonstrated the positive effect of predigested protein in stimulating pancreatic secretion and CCK release. Increased bicarbonate is also a huge advantage, as it provides the appropriate pH for pancreatic enzyme activity. Without that pH environment, digestive problems, gas, nutrient and protein deficiencies, and allergies result.

In people with celiac disease, CCK and gallbladder responses to oral or intestinal fats are abolished and intestinal CCK concentrations are greatly diminished. The cells that produce CCK are in the jejunal mucosa (the mucous membrane in the middle portion of the small intestine). In a study of six untreated celiac patients (ages 23–53), biopsies revealed an abnormal jejunal mucosa,[11] thought to be the reason why fats are not digested and CCK is not released. Intraduodenal administration of non-predigested fat did not induce any statistical change in blood CCK, whereas predigested fat evoked an immediate, significant increase, indicating that the jejunal mucosa can be prompted to produce CCK. Similarly, integrated gall-bladder contraction in response to predigested fat was significantly greater. These are crucial factors that can help celiac patients or anybody who is having problems digesting fats.

Predigested Foods Provide Better Protein Absorption

Proteins are the building blocks of muscle, blood, nails, skin, organs, hormones, antibodies, and much more. Amino acids, in turn, are the building blocks of proteins. Whole proteins are usually 50 or more amino acids linked together. During digestion, proteins are broken into smaller peptides (two or more amino acids linked together) and singular amino acids. Their eventual metabolism releases energy to drive cellular functioning. Without proper protein absorption, the list of potential health problems would be too long to fit in this book. So what's the best way to aid proper protein digestion and absorption?

Long-term supplementation with single amino acids (isolates) can cause protein imbalances, as they seem to compete with each other for absorption and are not absorbed in a consistent ratio—one can be absorbed faster than another, or more of one can enter the bloodstream than another, depending on the amounts taken. Peptides are often more bioavailable and more consistently absorbed than free amino acids.

Experiments have demonstrated that in predigested whole foods, both peptides and single amino acids must be present in the food mixture for optimum protein digestion. Evidence shows that protein is absorbed from the small intestine in the form of peptides as well as free amino acids, and that they aid each other and act as a transport system for proper absorption.

In one experiment, casein (a milk protein) was predigested by papain and other proteolytic enzymes into a mixture containing 50 percent free amino acids and about 50 percent small peptides. The compared mixture of free amino acids resembled the components of casein but was not predigested, nor did it contain peptides.[11]

These mixtures were introduced at separate times into the jejunum of six normal adult volunteers to observe their final digestion. The results showed considerable variation in the extent to which individual amino acids were absorbed from the amino acid mixture. For example, methionine (75 percent), leucine (51–59 percent), and isoleucine (50–59 percent) were well absorbed, whereas threonine (17 percent) and histidine (16 percent) were poorly absorbed.

Variation in absorption of amino acids from the predigested casein mixture was much less, and the amino acids that were poorly absorbed from the free amino acid mixture showed a tendency to be better absorbed from the predigested mixture. Seven amino acids (phenylalanine, alanine, tyrosine, serine, aspartic acid, threonine, and histidine) were absorbed to a greater extent from the predigested mixture.

Compared to the free amino acid mixture, protein absorption from the predigested mixture was 29 percent greater—a huge difference. In other words, 9 grams of predigested protein can equal 27 grams of a non-predigested protein mixture. People taking protein powders may not be absorbing proteins as well as they think! Plus, amino acid imbalances can create problems.

The finding that a number of amino acids were better absorbed from the predigested food gives evidence that peptides and free amino acids are a better source for protein absorption, and that eating predigested foods would be a better choice for people with digestive difficulties, for growing children, and especially for athletes. It's important not only that the overall absorption percentage is better, but also that when individual or free amino acids are taken, their absorption rates range from 70 percent to 16 percent, indicating competition for absorption. Peptides are necessary for proper amino acid transport through the intestinal wall into the bloodstream.

In a study at Central Middlesex Hospital, London,[16] several different protein foods were enzymatically predigested by papain and a mixture of pancreatic proteolytic enzymes and compared to their free amino acid counterparts. The foods were albumin (egg protein), lactalbumin (milk protein), and blends of casein/soy/lactalbumin and meat/soy lactalbumin. A double-lumen perfusion tube was inserted into the jejunum of 19 normal volunteers aged 20–27 years old.

In all cases, absorption of individual amino acids from the free amino acid mixtures varied considerably. In fact, phenylalanine, threonine, glutamic acid, and histidine were poorly absorbed from all of them. This marked difference was not observed with the predigested whole foods, from which amino acids were also absorbed significantly faster. Thirteen amino acids were absorbed faster from the casein/soy lactalbumin blend than the equivalent free amino acid mixture, and the meat/soy/lactalbumin blend had seven amino acids absorbed faster than its equivalent mixture.

Overall, regardless of the predigestion method, 29 percent of the total amino acids were absorbed faster than their equivalent free amino acid mixtures.

The wide variation in free amino acid uptake is attributed not only to their competition for absorption, but also to their reduced affinity for absorption in the absence of peptides that normally aid in their transport across the intestinal wall. The kinetic energy, motion, and absorption of amino acids are mediated by peptides in the solution, compared to free amino acid systems without peptides.

Researchers Y.S. Kim and E.J. Brophy have shown that mammalian intestines contain protein hydrolase enzymes, capable of hydrolyzing (breaking down) peptide chains.[17] The presence of hydrolases also indicates that for optimum digestion, it's natural to consume protein foods naturally predigested by their own enzymes into a mixture of peptides and free amino acids.

INTERACTING SYSTEMS IN BODY AND MIND

Interrelationship of Enzymes and the Immune System

When substances such as undigested protein, viruses, bacteria, fungi, toxins, or normal, everyday cellular wastes enter your bloodstream, your immune system reacts. These invaders are called antigens. Once the immune system identifies them, the bone marrow, spleen, and lymphatic system produce immunoglobulin proteins called antibodies, which are specific to each antigen. Specialized white blood cells called lymphocytes release the antibodies, which attach themselves to their antigens like a lock and key, or like holding hands. Antibodies connected to their "trapped" antigens, called circulating immune complexes (CICs), stimulate scavenger immune system cells called macrophages to destroy, "swallow," and remove the offenders. This is detoxification.

Normally, CICs are easily eliminated from the body and no problem ensues. But if these complexes become excessive, they can interfere with functions such as nutrient and hormonal absorption and the transportation of bodily fluids. The presence of CICs in autoimmune diseases, inflammatory disorders, heart disease, and cancer has been scientifically documented; overabundant CICs can actually act as an immunosuppressant. Here's where enzymes come to the rescue. Enzymes such as pancreatin, trypsin, lipase, amylase, and papain can break up CICs and also inhibit the formation of new immune complexes.

All cells have receptor sites, or "docking stations," on their membranes. Hormones and other substances dock at these sites and can then enter the cell. For a cell to be healthy and carry on its functions, its docking stations need to be clear. Toxic CICs can be deposited on the cell's surface, blocking these sites. Proteolytic enzymes have been shown to alter these complexes and free the cell from such deposits. Studies have also shown a decrease in CICs after oral administration of enzyme combinations. In this way, enzymes demonstrate a regulatory and stimulatory effect on the immune system.

I want to explain what I mean by "regulatory." One form of communication within the body is through the release and reception of hormones called cytokines. There are many types of cytokines for conveying various messages to cells. For example, if a virus has invaded, the whole body gets the message by way of cytokine release and circulation throughout the bloodstream. But if cells are toxic and their docking sites are blocked, the messages they receive get distorted. Proteolytic enzymes have been shown to help regulate this function of the cytokine transport system. These important, far-reaching effects of enzymes in our bodies are a most overlooked subject in the health industry.

There is a connection between the strength of our immune system and our enzyme level. The greater the enzyme reserve, the stronger our immune system, the healthier and stronger we will be. It has been clearly stated that enzyme activity increases during digestion and also during any other increase in metabolism, such as that in acute disease. But what is the exact relationship between our immune system and enzymes?

Leukocytes (white blood cells) are responsible for destroying foreign, disease-producing substances in the blood and lymph fluids. During acute disease and infection, the white blood cell count increases to help fight off these pathologies.

Dr. Willstatter, in an early enzyme study, found eight different amylases in leukocytes and noted a remarkably close correspondence between the enzyme systems of the leukocytes and the pancreas.[40] Investigations have also shown that leukocytes contain proteolytic and lipolytic enzymes very similar to those secreted by the pancreas. Given that these enzymes are found in the leukocytes and that the leukocytes transport these throughout the body, it seems that the pancreas (and most likely, other enzyme-secreting glands) receives a significant amount of enzymes from leukocytes.

These enzymes act very much like the enzymes in our digestive tract, as they break down undigested proteins, fats, and carbohydrates that have been absorbed by the blood and could cause problems if not eliminated. Enzymes act as scavengers in the body, latching onto foreign substances and reducing them to a disposable form. They also prevent arteries from clogging up and joints from becoming gummed up.

It was once thought that the pancreas produced all of these enzymes, but as mentioned earlier, this idea is erroneous. As small as the pancreas is, it couldn't possibly produce all the enzymes found in the muscles, glands, and tissues, as well as those used daily in digestion and those lost through the sweat, urine, and feces. As it turns out, enzymes are produced by all the tissues of the body. And it's been shown that the enzymes of white blood cells act very much like the enzymes of the pancreas, especially the proteolytic enzymes.

During acute disease, body enzyme levels rise, whereas during chronic disease, enzyme levels are decreased. The pancreas and digestive tract are weakened, for example, in diabetes, cancer, and chronic intestinal problems. During the course of a chronic disease, the immune system also shows signs of great expenditure. The correlation is clear: enzymes are related to all diseases, whether acute or chronic, via the immune system.

Our enzyme levels must be maintained at any expense to help maintain vitality and endurance and to prevent disease. If pancreatic enzyme output is hindered, the whole body is affected. If disease is present, enzymes are used up to fight the condition, and the pancreas is overworked. You can see how eating mostly cooked food all our lives, or trying to overcome a chronic disease while still eating this type of diet, can be detrimental.

Blood Sugar and the Brain

It seems that our happiness depends largely upon the thoughts we think, but it is impossible to think positively at all times when we are toxic, stiff, and experiencing low blood sugar levels. Our brain subsists exclusively on large amounts of sugar (in the form of glucose) and oxygen. When this supply is low, we experience a lack of concentration, insomnia, lethargy, irritability, and confusion.

A lack of enzymes, oxygen, and sugar supplies to the cells of our body can cause hypoglycemia. Hypoglycemia is a disorder resulting from excessively low blood sugar, the primary fuel for our cells. Authorities have estimated that anywhere from *ten to 100 million Americans* suffer from hypoglycemia.

Because hypoglycemia is a malfunction of our fuel supply, every organ is affected. As the sugar level drops, the metabolism of every organ drops, resulting in fatigue and psychosomatic problems. Because the brain depends on glucose, a drop in one's blood sugar can cause mental fatigue and depression.

The endocrine glands—especially the pituitary, adrenals, thyroid, and pancreas—control the blood sugar level. Here's how:

- The pancreas secretes insulin, which decreases blood sugar by facilitating the movement of glucose from the bloodstream into the cells. Insulin also stimulates liver and muscle cells to convert glucose into glycogen, which is the chief stored form of sugar in the body.

- The adrenal glands secrete the hormone epinephrine to prompt the breakdown of stored glycogen back into glucose, which then enters the bloodstream to raise blood sugar.

- Meanwhile, the thyroid gland secretes hormones that control the rate at which the body uses oxygen, as well as hormones that increase the rate of energy released from carbohydrates.

- All of these glands are controlled by the pituitary gland, which, in turn, is controlled by an area of the brain called the hypothalamus. The hypothalamus receives information from all parts of the body via the nervous system. This information includes emotional state, body temperature, and blood nutrient concentration, among many other things. The endocrine system and the nervous system also cooperate to regulate the appetite.

It has been shown that the pituitary and other glands can enlarge, become exhausted, and be susceptible to disease when an enzyme deficiency exists. If blood amylase is lacking, blood sugar levels can be higher than normal; blood sugar levels have been lowered by administering amylase. Investigators Deichmann-Grubler and Myers demonstrated that giving amylase preparations to normal individuals who had eaten 80 grams of glucose maintained their blood sugar level.[11]

Reports show that oral or intravenous administration of amylase lowers blood sugar levels in diabetics. In one study, 86 percent of the examined diabetics had amylase-deficient intestinal secretions; after amylase was given to a majority of these patients, 50 percent of those who had previously been insulin-dependent could control their blood sugar without insulin.[33] Amylase seems to help the storage and utilization of sugar in the bloodstream.

Cooked food, in which amylase and other enzymes are destroyed, has a tremendous effect on blood sugar levels. A study at George Washington University Hospital examined the effects of eating raw and cooked starch. As illustrated in Diagram 4, when 50 grams of raw starch were fed to the patients, blood sugar increased an average of 1 milligram per 100 cubic centimeters in ½-hour, decreased 1.2 milligrams in 1 hour, and decreased 3 milligrams in 2 hours. After 50 grams of cooked starch, the average blood sugar increase was 56 milligrams in ½-hour, then a drop to 51 milligrams in 1 hour, and then down to 11 milligrams in 2 hours.[10]

Notice the difference between the blood sugar responses to cooked versus raw starch (raw starch has enzymes in it). Blood sugar after eating cooked starch rose to 56 milligrams in ½-hour, as opposed to the mere 1-milligram rise with uncooked starch. After 2 hours, the cooked-starch blood sugar level fell to 11 milligrams—a 45-milligram drop—which resulted in fatigue, anxiety, and the other afore-mentioned symptoms. By contrast, the raw-starch blood sugar level only showed a drop of 1–3 milligrams in 2 hours, and that group experienced a much steadier metabolic rate and emotional stability.

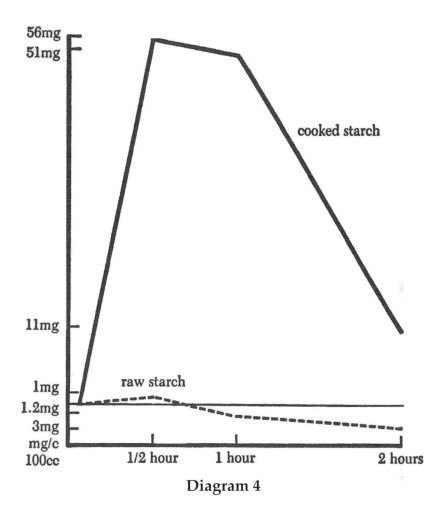

Diagram 4

The endocrine glands need minerals and vitamins from properly digested food and/or supplements to function effectively; for example, the thyroid needs iodine, and the adrenals need vitamin C. As you know, overcooked food is deficient not only in enzymes but also in other nutrients, and these deficiencies can cause many problems.

The glands are stimulated by the brain to secrete their hormones. When blood sugar level drops below normal, the pancreas and adrenals are prompted to secrete their hormones. When the blood is lacking the nutrients that support the endocrine glands, the hypothalamus stimulates the appetite and causes a craving for food. The more cooked food is eaten, the more the hormones stimulate appetite and cravings, resulting in overeating—and excessive eating, of course, can cause you to become overweight or even obese. (Obesity can then lead to heart problems, high blood pressure, and many other diseases.) Quick rising and falling blood sugar levels in the body cause emotional swings and mental imbalances. Finally, the endocrine glands, deficient in their secretions from trying to normalize the body's metabolism, become exhausted. This state can be the foundation of both mental and physical diseases.

Enzymes and Mental Health

Enzymes have as much to do with our physical and mental health as any other element of nutrition. This subject has not been given enough attention. Usually, we don't look at our brain the same way as we look at the rest of our body. It needs nutrients to survive and function properly. The brain either controls or produces more than 60 neurotransmitters. Anxiety, panic attacks, and social anxiety disorder can all be helped by digestive enzymes and improved nutrition.

A good example of this is using an amino acid called tryptophan to increase serotonin in the brain. Serotonin is a calming, relaxing neurotransmitter that relieves anxiety, panic, and depression. At night, serotonin is released in the brain and puts you to sleep. I once had my amino acids measured by a blood test, and my tryptophan level was so low, I couldn't believe it. After taking tryptophan for a few months, my serotonin level went back to normal; I sleep great now, and my fear of flying is totally gone. (For more information on amino acids, hormones, and neurotransmitters, see my book *ProMetabolics: Your Personal Guide to Transformational Health and Healing*.)

The point I'm making is that without good digestion and the proper enzyme mix, these mental problems can exist. And most of them are caused by nutritional deficiencies.

Another good example is low blood sugar, which, as mentioned, stems from a lack of amylase—basically, all blood sugar problems do. Blood sugar can form high triglycerides in the bloodstream, resulting in a clumping of blood, or "blood sludge," that thickens the blood and thereby inhibits circulation of hormones and nutrients. All of this is due to poor digestion. Dr. Melvyn Werbach, in *Nutritional Influences on Illness: A Sourcebook of Clinical Research*, states, "It is well known that certain nutritional deficiencies can produce schizophrenia and psychoses."[38] (Additional books available on this subject include *Brain Fitness* by Dr. Goldman, *Your Miracle Brain* by Jean Carper, and *Healing the Mind the Natural Way* by Pat Lazarus. Please don't think there's no help; it's all out there for the reading.)

Nutritional Recommendations for Mental Health

My suggested program for mental health uses digestive enzymes as the foundational supplement, along with a complete amino acid supplement, a whole-food drink or supplement like Juice Plus+®, and the essential omega 3, 6, and 9 fatty acids. Consult a good nutritional therapist and see where else you may be deficient. Make sure your enzyme product is plant-derived and contains all four categories of digestive enzymes: lipase, amylase, protease, and cellulase.

How can we be mentally "on top" and face the world around us if we can't think straight? A deficient brain is a deficient mind. I just made that up! Stay mentally well.

AGING AND LONGEVITY

Dr. Howell states, "Enzymes are a true yardstick of vitality. Enzymes offer an important means of calculating the vital energy of an organism. That which we call energy, vital force, nerve energy, and strength, may be synonymous with enzyme activity."[11]

The buildup and breakdown of tissues is performed by enzymes. In other words, enzyme activity maintains your metabolism and determines its rate of speed. The more rapid the metabolic process, the more enzymes are required to participate, and thus, the faster enzymes are used up. When your enzyme level is lowered, your metabolism is lowered, and so is your energy level. Don't misunderstand—I'm not saying that enzymes are the source of life, but that a strong correlation exists between an organism's enzyme level, its energy level, and the youth of its tissues.

At the University of Toronto, a team of scientists showed that life runs its course in direct proportion to the catabolic rate.[11] Catabolic rate is a measure of the rapidity of the wear and tear on the body, or the rate of tissue breakdown. It corresponds to the aging process. And as you know, this tissue breakdown is performed by enzymes. Therefore, the faster the breakdown, the more enzymes are used up. Our enzyme reserve can be used up rapidly, or it can be preserved. Taking enzyme supplements and eating raw foods are ways to add enzymes to our reserve and add to our energy level.

Why We Age

There have been many theories of aging, from genetic theories to all sorts of ideas on how our DNA and tissues change during the aging process. I see a huge problem with most of them: when we examine a tissue's change, we're studying the result, not the causative factor. If a tissue, organ, or cell has changed in some fashion, what caused it? The cause is always before the effect. These physical changes are not the cause—the cause lies deeper.

We exhaust our enzyme levels as we get older, as I have discussed. Most disease starts with a type of insult or injury to the body; then we see the result—inflammation. If we have an enzyme deficiency, our immune system can't put the fire out. Blood clots and fibrin build up in the areas of insult without enough proteolytic enzymes to dissolve them. How we damage our bodies (the cause) has to be eliminated; then we have to use enzymes to reduce the inflammation (the effect).

Prevention is the best cure. To prevent, we must have the knowledge to avoid most of the environmental and dietary abuses and errors that weaken our immunity and cause premature aging. The first proactive approach to slowing aging is to preserve your bodily enzymes. We should take hold of this opportunity with both hands.

We Age by the Second

Every normal molecule in your body has electrons spinning in pairs in its outer orbit. These paired electrons keep the molecule in perfect balance and acting in a very specific way according to its nature. If a molecule gains or loses one of these paired outer electrons for any reason, it becomes imbalanced and unstable—it is now a free radical. Unpaired electrons seek other electrons to pair with. Thus, free radicals are reactive, and they attack other molecules. That's one of the main ways free radicals damage our tissues: by stealing electrons from the molecules in cell membranes, weakening the affected cells.

Free radicals can be found anywhere in the body. Wherever excess free radical activity destroys cells faster than the body can replace them, tissue death or even organ death occurs. Excess free radicals are the direct result of chemical exposure, emotional stress, exercise, sunlight, smoking, radiation, and drugs. And in addition to these outside agents and special conditions, free radicals are generated by the body. An adult body at rest can produce 4 pounds of free radicals a year—and if exposed to smoke, other environmental toxins, and exercise, it can produce up to 20 pounds a year.

One type of free radical results from energy production by the mitochondria during normal cellular metabolism. Mitochondria are the "tiny furnaces" in each cell. Essentially, they combine oxygen with food—proteins, carbohydrates, and fats—to convert these nutrients into energy, in the form of ATP molecules. This oxidation process also releases free radicals. Some of the most common free radicals produced by the body are superoxide, hydroxyl, and hydrogen peroxide, and these are responsible for considerable damage. On top of those, smoking, drugs, and other chemicals bring their own free radicals into the picture, adding to what you've already produced.

The ultimate achievement for free radicals is to establish stability, either by transferring electrons to another atom or molecule or grabbing electrons from another atom or molecule. In either case, a free radical achieves stability only by creating another one, which then prowls the body, seeking stable atoms or molecules for electron transfer or stripping, and so on. This chain reaction can have disastrous consequences: for instance, it's been calculated that a single free radical can damage about 26 molecules of polyunsaturated fat before losing its momentum.[28] The destruction of unsaturated fats in cell membranes and the bloodstream is one of the most damaging effects of free radicals.

Cross-Linkage: Aging Tissues

At the tissue level, free radical damage is called cross-linkage. Cross-linkages are particular bonds connecting the amino acid chains in proteins. Some cross-linkage is normal, but abnormal cross-linkage indicates aging. The most obvious external sign of cross-linkage is our skin's loss of elasticity, leading to wrinkles, stiffness, and sagging. Decreased enzyme activity and increased cross-linkage also give rise to age spots (lipofuscin) and blemishes.

Eighty percent of our skin is connective tissue, which provides strength and elasticity. Connective tissue made of giant protein chains connects the whole body. Like the mesh on a trampoline or the strings on a violin, these protein chains are normally connected in such a way that they don't restrict each other. If they were tied together, or cross-linked, they wouldn't stretch or vibrate as they're supposed to.

Free radicals, too much sun, poor diet, pesticides, radiation, nicotine, and more can all cause this problem. The DNA and RNA strands in our genes can also be damaged and cross-linked. Think of a lifetime of cross-linkage in all the types of protein in your body, and you'll get a sense of what aging is all about. The affected tissues become dysfunctional and interfere with circulation and nutrient and hormonal transport. (And what good is taking hormones or supplements if they can't reach the intended tissue sites?)

Diagram 5 depicts normal collagen protein and overly cross-linked collagen protein. Three amino acid chains twisted together form each collagen unit. In youth, there's only a small amount of cross-linkage between the units (top of diagram). With increasing age, more cross-linkage occurs (bottom of diagram). The result is less-elastic connective tissue.

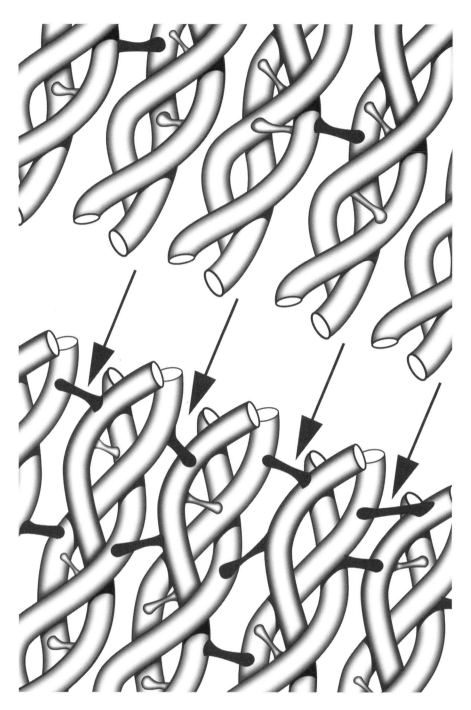

Diagram 5 (Illustration by Eric Lindley.)

Enzymes and Other Antioxidants Are Aging Antidotes

But don't despair, because your body has a natural defense against free radicals: antioxidants. The antioxidants you produce are the enzymes superoxide dismutase, catalase, and glutathione peroxidase. Enzymes bind to connective tissue and help to break up cross-linkage and improve circulation. They also neutralize free radicals, which can then be disposed of harmlessly. Antioxidant supplements in addition to enzymes can be taken to assist an anti-aging regime—vitamins A, C, and E, zinc, selenium, proteolytic enzymes such as bromelain and papain, and Juice Plus+®, for example. However, your primary antioxidant source is— or should be—a diet high in fruits and vegetables.

Enzymes and Longevity

Studying the comparative enzyme content of blood, urine, and digestive fluids in the human population has generated some very important data. It's been shown that young adults have a high potential enzyme reserve in their tissues, whereas in older persons' tissues, the potential enzyme reserve is much lower—essentially, depleted. In an experiment at the Michael Reese Hospital in Chicago, a comparison of salivary amylase between young adults (aged 21–31) and older adults (aged 69–100) showed the younger group had 30 times more amylase in their saliva than the older group.[11]

When a young person eats cooked food, there is a greater outpouring of enzymes from the organs and body fluids than in an adult. This is because years of eating a cooked-food diet with only a fraction of its original enzyme content has depleted the adult's enzyme reserve, whereas the young adult's reserve is still high. The higher amount of enzymes is why younger people can tolerate a diet of white bread, starches, and predominantly cooked food. However, as enzyme reserves decline over the years, these same foods can cause illnesses such as constipation, blood diseases, bleeding ulcers, bloating, and arthritis. In older individuals, the body's enzyme content has been bankrupted and these kinds of foods are not properly digested. Instead, they ferment in the digestive tract, producing toxins that are then absorbed into the blood and deposited in the joints and other tissues.

During chronic disease, the enzyme content in blood, urine, feces, and tissues is reduced, whereas in acute disease (and sometimes at the beginning of chronic disease), the enzyme content is often found to be high. This shows that the body's reserve is not yet depleted; consequently, an outpouring of enzymes can join in the battle against disease. But as the disease progresses, the body's enzyme content is lowered.

This parallel between diminished enzymes during chronic disease and old age is often misunderstood. A low enzyme content in old age is often looked upon as normal, whereas a low content during chronic disease is considered pathological. The truth is that age is not so much a matter of chronology, but rather of integrity of the body's tissues. Every cell in these tissues depends upon the amount of enzymes present to carry on its metabolism. There is a definite correlation between an individual's amount of enzymes and amount of energy. Increasing age causes a slow decrease in enzyme reserves, metabolism suffers as the enzyme level becomes low, and death is the final result.

Hazards of Excess Food and Excess Protein

At Brown University, a group of 158 overfed animals lived an average of 29.6 days, while another group on a starvation diet (small amounts of food and fluid) lived an average of 39.19 days—an increased longevity of about 40 percent.[13] At the very least, this should make us look at our own food intake and determine if we are indeed over-ingesting.

A high-protein diet is very stimulating to the body but can cause serious damage. When the diet contains more protein than is needed, the excess is broken down by enzymes in the liver and kidneys. The major by-product of protein breakdown is urea, a diuretic, which stimulates the kidneys to produce more urine. One of the most important minerals lost through urine is calcium. When the participants in one experiment consumed 75 grams of protein daily, even with a concurrent calcium intake as high as 1,400 milligrams, they lost more calcium through urine than they'd actually absorbed from what they took in.[25] In such cases, the deficit must be made up by the body's calcium reserve, which is taken from the bones. Mineral-deficient bones, in turn, are a steppingstone to osteoporosis.

The aforementioned experiments show that when excessive protein, or food in general, is eaten, there is a corresponding decrease in enzyme, vitamin, and mineral levels. Similarly, when the metabolism is artificially increased by coffee or other stimulants, enzymes are used up and a false energy output is experienced. Although you may feel a sense of well-being, the end result will be *lower* energy, more rapid enzyme burnout, and premature old age.

INFLAMMATION, DISEASE, AND ALLERGY

Enzymes, the circulatory system, the nervous system, the endocrine system, and the digestive system are connected and interdependent in all life processes. Disease rarely involves just one or two organs—usually the entire body is affected. In natural therapeutics, all diseases are considered to be systemic problems. This means that all body processes are involved. To bring about favorable results, the whole body must be influenced in a positive direction.

When cooked food or unnatural substances are eaten, the body is depleted of enzymes, minerals, vitamins, and amino acids. No one can afford this sustained depletion. Gradually, as we lose nutrients, our body processes begin to weaken. Fatigue is one of the first signs; finally, sickness results. This is the disease process. But many physicians encountering a sickness seem to believe that disease is both the cause and the effect.

Chronic diseases sometimes take years to develop, and poor nutrition has been estimated to cause a third of all our sicknesses. In the last several years, intense research has gotten physicians and the public worldwide to realize that what we feed our bodies has everything to do with the cause and treatment of illness. The importance of enzymes cannot be overemphasized. If a lack of enzymes can cause disease, then adding enzymes to the diet by supplementation and/or proper food can help to prevent and treat it. Considering that enzymes are used up daily, replacing them is the logical thing to do.

Understanding Inflammation

According to Drs. Wolf and Ransberger, "Inflammation in its multitude of forms is perhaps the most general and fundamental reaction in all pathological processes."[41] If you understand this process and learn how to control it with enzymes and nutrition, you can halt almost any disease. From a common cold to cancer, the inflammatory process is present in all disease. These are powerful statements. In spite of the extreme differences in location and cause between urinary infections, measles, sunburn, hepatitis, burns, arthritis, allergies, heart disease, and viral infections, the body's biochemical process relating to inflammation is principally the same.

Inflammation is denoted by any word ending in "itis." In immediate response to any insult or injury to the body, be it chemical (toxic), physical, microbial, or due to another foreign substance, a three-stage series of defense measures starts: the reaction phase, the repair phase, and finally the regeneration phase. During each phase, diet, herbs, enzymes, and drugs can be used for support. (My book *Natural Healing with Herbs* covers cleansing, building, and tonification therapies, among others.) You've likely heard, for example, that echinacea and vitamin C reduce inflammation. Here, I'm going to focus on the use of enzymes for that purpose.

At the moment of insult/injury, the reaction phase starts with the aim of preventing the harm or damage from spreading. The body tries to isolate the focal point and restore normal physiology (metabolism) as soon as possible. The reactions of heat, redness, pain, fever, swelling, and edema are all secondary symptoms of the inflammatory process, conveying information about the changes taking place. The use of steroids and nonsteroidal drugs can stop or interfere with this healing process.

Cells and tiny blood vessels begin to discharge pus and other fluids from the injury, and white blood cells gather in the area of the focal point. These white blood cells engulf germs or damaged tissue and enclose the area by projecting a protein-like film, stopping the inflammation from spreading. The injured area is walled off as an area for healing, or the repair phase.

The white blood cells use clotting substances (semi-solid gel) to seal off inflamed areas and enclose toxins. Among these substances are fibrin, a stringy, insoluble protein, which is formed from another blood protein, fibrinogen. This is the beginning of the acute inflammatory changes in tissue, as the fibrin mesh also interferes with circulation at the focus of inflammation. That's how the pain, redness, and swelling are caused.

So this part of the repair phase is a double-edged sword. To focus healing on the area inflammation, it must be contained, but that slows circulation, which must be restored after the healing is finished. But if we do not take care of our body's needs, these focal areas become chronically inflamed, and the disease process begins. Fibromyalgia and arthritis are perfect examples.

Proteolytic Enzymes in Inflammation and Healing

As you now know, proteolytic enzymes break down protein substances. In digestion, they break down protein foods; in inflammation, they exhibit their miraculous activity at the focus area. During the formation of fibrin, proteolytic enzymes secreted by leukocytes begin breaking the fibrin down into smaller amino acids, to inhibit the buildup of any more than is needed for healing. Fibrin's function in the body is thereby kept in balance by proteolytic enzymes.

You can see how intelligent the body is. A building-up and breaking-down process takes place until the inflammatory focus is healed and normal circulation resumes. Basically, all three phases (reaction, repair, and regeneration) happen at roughly the same time, and overlap—it's just that one phase is more dominant at any given time. Proteolytic enzymes are secreted in all three.

Trypsin, papain, and bromelain can be taken orally at the onset of inflammation. When these enzymes are used preventatively, fibrin deposits are limited, and healing is accelerated. These and other proteolytic enzymes have been used in therapy for nearly all inflammatory diseases. Athletes can take them before workouts to limit injuries and inflammation. (I take them before every workout.) They also can be taken at the beginning of colds, fever, and flu. What a healthful way to assist your body!

Test and Natural Countermeasures for Inflammation

One way to find out the extent of inflammation is to test for C-reactive protein. C-reactive protein is produced in the liver by inflammatory cytokines. The presence of too much of this marker indicates an increased risk for atherosclerotic plaque and abnormal blood clotting. Such plaques can block the blood flow in a coronary artery, resulting in a heart attack. Some studies show that people with high levels of C-reactive protein are almost three times more likely to have a heart attack. C-reactive protein can be suppressed by supplemental DHEA, vitamins E and K, fish oil, and nettle leaf extract.

High levels of the same coagulating fibrinogen that so helpfully turns into fibrin to promote healing can also induce heart attacks by thickening the blood and increasing platelet aggregation. You need enough fibrinogen to heal, but not so much that it creates another problem. This is another scenario in which proteolytic enzymes play a part, by liquefying fibrinogen. Aspirin, green tea, ginkgo, vitamin E, and garlic also help to thin the blood and prevent unnecessary coagulation.

Enzyme Levels in Disease

When certain enzymes are found in excess, they can indicate specific disease states. For example, the pancreas normally secretes a large amount of the fat-digesting enzyme lipase—much of it drawn from the blood—into the digestive tract. Thus, an elevated blood lipase level can point specifically to pancreatic disease, as serum lipase levels rise when pancreatic inflammation occurs. As another example, the enzyme acid phosphatase, which breaks down phosphates in the bloodstream, is found in the prostate gland, red blood cells, and platelets. In these locations, blood serum enzyme levels are measured primarily to evaluate the possible presence of prostatic carcinoma (a malignant growth).

In acute diseases (and during exercise), the body's overall enzyme level increases. In 1933, Dr. Gerner measured 300 amylase levels in 115 patients with 28 different acute infectious diseases, and found that urinary amylase was increased in 73 percent of the entire group. During pneumonia, acute appendicitis, malaria, pulmonary tuberculosis, fevers of all types, and children's diseases, he found enzymes were elevated in the blood, urine, and feces.[11]

Any increase in metabolic activity, whether it is associated with fever, heart action, digestion, muscular work, or pregnancy, is paralleled by an increase in enzyme activity. Enzyme activity increases as temperatures increase, as in most acute disease conditions and during exercise. Enzymes perform more work during fevers of 104°F than at normal body temperatures. It is therefore evident that if enzymes respond to fever and infection, they have a direct relationship to our body's defense mechanisms. Similarly, when fevers are reduced, so is the enzyme activity.

A chronic disease, having lingered for many weeks, months, or even years, has been a constant drag on the body, depleting its vitamins and minerals. During chronic disease processes, there is usually a low body reserve of enzymes as well. For example, in a studied group of 111 tuberculosis patients, 82 percent had lower enzyme levels than normal individuals, and as the disease worsened, the levels decreased further.[11] In diabetic patients, Dr. Volodin found that enzyme levels in the urine, blood, and intestines were usually decreased, along with decreased pancreatic lipase and trypsin in five of six patients, and with feces also indicating incomplete digestion of meat and fats.[11] With skin afflictions such as psoriasis, dermatitis, and pruritis, Dr. Ottenstein found low blood amylase.[11] In another interesting experiment involving 40 patients with liver diseases such as cirrhosis, hepatitis, and cholecystitis (gallbladder inflammation), their blood amylase was low, and when the blood amylase level rose, both their general condition and liver condition improved.[9]

The overall evidence that enzymes are used more rapidly during disease, detoxification, and digestion (every time metabolism speeds up) highlights the importance of supporting our enzyme reserves at all times. As Dr. Howell puts it, "When we eat cooked enzyme-free food, the body is forced to produce enzymes needed for digestion. This depletes the body's limited enzyme capacity. This stealing of enzymes from other parts of the body sets up a competition for enzymes among the various organs and tissues in the body. The resulting metabolic dislocations may be the cause of cancer, heart disease, diabetes, and many other chronic incurable diseases."[10]

Remember, all inflammatory conditions go through the same phases. A program to prevent inflammatory conditions is foundational; then you can get specific with the rest of your herbal, nutritional, and drug program to meet your individual needs. I suggest you work with the guidance and supervision of a skilled therapist. (See *ProMetabolics: Your Personal Guide to Transformation Health and Healing*, for a self-monitoring system that tells you exactly "where you're at" during any health condition, and how to support your body.)

Inflammation and Cross-Linkage in Circulatory and Heart Disease

Inflammation manifests in circulatory and heart disease. In 1997, a very large study showed that aspirin (an anti-inflammatory drug) helped to lower the risk of heart disease and stroke in a group of 22,000 men.[24,31] Unfortunately, long-term use of aspirin—even buffered aspirin—leads to significant gastrointestinal complications, including micro-bleeding, ulcers, and upsetting your natural bacterial balance. What such studies demonstrate, however, is that curbing inflammation is at "the heart" of a cardiovascular wellness program.

The gradual closure of our arteries is a principle cause of death. Stroke, atherosclerosis, circulatory disease, and thrombosis are all degrees of the same thing. As you've seen, proteolytic enzymes can control the buildup of fibrin in the blood; they also limit the production of immune complexes. These aging and disease processes can be somewhat controlled by improving our lifestyle, and the same goes for circulatory diseases.

Dr. Johan Bjorksten at the Research Foundation, Madison, WI, describes cross-linkage in blood vessels.[3] The vessels' inner walls (intima) are exposed to circulating cross-linked molecules, especially if enzymes are deficient and therefore not available to break up these cross-linked molecules for elimination. Arteries gradually lose elasticity, a primary effect of cross-linkage. The walls harden, weaken, and become permeable, so blood plasma leaks through them. As the body tries to heal these areas, immune system cells gather and collagen can form, hindering blood flow. The resulting ingrowth of tissue can block the vessel.

Enzymes for the Circulatory System

A significant amount of medical evidence supports the use of enzymes to improve cardiovascular and circulatory health, phlebitis, edema, varicose veins, and other conditions affecting the heart, lungs, kidneys, and liver. We finally have a safe anti-inflammatory tool: one of the most researched enzyme mixtures today is a product called Wobenzym®, from Germany (available through Mountain State Health Products; www.mhpvitamins.com). Wobenzym® has been proven to lower the bloodstream's C-reactive protein significantly.[22]

But enzymes go beyond just balancing C-reactive protein. By breaking down excessive fibrinogen, they've been proven to reduce blood clotting and inflammation and to substantially improve circulation throughout the body.[41] In one study, Dr. Valls-Serra treated 245 patients with enzymes and demonstrated their effectiveness at reducing blood clotting in thrombophlebitis (vein inflammation involving the formation of blood clots).[11]

When taking enzymes therapeutically, you always want them to be absorbed directly into the bloodstream, so it's important to take them between meals to prevent their diversion into the digestive process. If you have heart or circulatory problems, pay special attention to the enzyme lipase. Lipase hydrolyzes fats (such as triglycerides) into monoglycerides and fatty acids; it is also involved in fat burning for energy and in the body's fat storage and distribution. It is found in high amounts in avocadoes, olives, seeds, nuts, and raw butter—basically, any naturally high-fat foods—and in medium amounts in some fruits such as cherries, bananas, and figs. You can take lipase between meals to help break down fats and fatty accumulations that cause congestive problems.

Lipase, Circulatory Disease, and Obesity

Enzyme deficiencies—in particular, lipase deficiency—can cause circulatory disease, high blood pressure, and other blood vessel problems. In certain areas of the body, they can also be a major factor in obesity. It has been reported that in human obesity, the lipase content of fatty tissue is decreased. Dr. David Galton of Tufts University School of Medicine examined 11 individuals weighing 230–240 pounds and found enzyme deficiencies in their fatty tissue—even their fatty tumors (lipomas) were deficient in lipase.[10] Animal tissues normally contain sizeable amounts of lipase. Why would this deficiency occur?

Many experiments have shown that when food is cooked, the lipase is absent. Some high-calorie foods such as meat and potatoes have high enzyme values when raw. Of course, many such foods are not eaten in their raw state. Unfortunately, when cooked, these same foods provide few, if any, enzymes. Without lipase, any overabundance of cooked calories is stored in the body as fat, which accumulates in the liver, kidneys, arteries, and capillaries.

The stress caused by enzyme-free food not only increases body weight, but also alters internal organs. For example, a heat-treated, refined-food diet lacking enzymes drastically changes the size and appearance of the pituitary gland. Conversely, surgical removal of glands in animals leads to changes in blood enzyme levels.[10] Enzymes affect hormone-producing glands, and hormones influence enzyme levels.

The secretions of the pancreas and pituitary are exhausted by the overstimulation of a cooked-food diet. Thyroid function also becomes exhausted, the body becomes sluggish, and the person gains weight. Raw calories, on the other hand, are relatively nonstimulating to glands and help to stabilize body weight. For example, when farmers feed raw potatoes to hogs, the hogs don't get fat, but feeding them cooked potatoes produces rapid weight gain (and more profit).[10] Think of the meat on the grocery shelves from animals like these, with high fat and low enzymes (even lower when cooked)—this fat is saturated, which makes it difficult to digest, and it accumulates in our arteries.

Fat, when not digested properly by lipase, can be absorbed in an adulterated state. This fat is later found in the blood vessels and arteries, causing conditions such as arteriosclerosis, high blood pressure, and high cholesterol. Fatty deposits clog the vessels and impede blood from reaching the heart, which can result in heart attack. The heart must work harder to push the blood through congested vessels—causing high blood pressure and an enlarged heart. The offenders in these problems are:

- saturated fats (particularly from animal products)
- hydrogenated fats
- polyunsaturated fats

We've all been told that polyunsaturated fats lower cholesterol levels. This is true, but they work like a drug. As stated in a fine book titled *The McDougall Plan*, "Poly-unsaturated vegetable oils can be a health hazard. When consumed, they act like a cholesterol-lowering drug. They drive large amounts of stored cholesterol from the body tissues through the liver to the gallbladder and into the colon. In the bowel, the excreted cholesterol may be involved in the cause of cancer of the colon."[25] (Rats fed diets high in cholesterol and polyunsaturated fat have more colon cancer than rats fed cholesterol and saturated fat.)

As you've learned, it has been shown that younger people have a higher enzyme content in their blood and tissues than older folks. Drs. Berker and Meyers, for instance, showed that the blood of a group of 77-year-olds had only half the lipase as the blood of a group of 27-year-olds. Their investigations also found deficient lipase in individuals who had arteriosclerosis (hardening of the arteries), high blood pressure, and slow fat absorption.[11] Researchers at Stanford University similarly showed that patients with arteriosclerosis were lipase-deficient in lipase; the more advanced the disease, the more enzyme-deficient the patient.[25] In another study demonstrating deficient blood enzymes in patients with arteriosclerosis, lipase was given to patients with slow fat metabolism and blood-fat problems, and their fat metabolism immediately improved.[25]

Fats in the bloodstream impair the function of the immune system's white blood cells by slowing circulation. This may be the reason why obese individuals seem to be infection-prone. High levels of fat in the blood also block the action of insulin, the hormone that regulates tissues' absorption of sugar; this interference causes blood sugar levels to rise, which can be a contributing factor in the development of diabetes.

Overfeeding and Weight Gain

Dr. G. E. Burch of Tulane University demonstrated some interesting findings related to the cause of obesity. He showed that young, overfed animals develop more fat cells than underfed ones.[10] Infants who are overfed can develop three times as many fat cells as is normal. When a normal person gains weight, he or she may get what is called "pleasingly plump," but when a person who has been overfed as an infant and who has accumulated many more fat cells has these cells filled to excess, obesity results. Both types of people can eat the same amount of food, but the one with more existing fat cells puts on weight much more easily. A good way to help these people is to add raw foods to their diet along with enzyme supplements. I lost 70 pounds doing exactly this, and by limiting my diet to mostly raw foods, I haven't gained a pound in 12 years.

If you want to reduce your weight and keep it down, eating fewer meals per day will be beneficial. Frequent eating and snacking can decrease the enzyme level of the body and cause weight gain. In an experiment carried out with two test groups of rats, one fed every 2 hours and the other fed once a day, the rats that ate once a day lived 17 percent longer, had lower body weight, and showed higher enzyme activity in their pancreas and fat cells.[10] (This experiment also found that enzyme activity in the tissues became weaker as the rats aged.)

Raw-Meat Diet?

Why is there such a high incidence of circulatory disease in "civilized" nations, and not in "uncivilized" groups of people? Primitive Eskimos, who consume as much as 10 pounds of raw fish and meat and blubber daily, don't develop vascular disease, because most of their food is raw. The enzymes—in particular, lipase—are still active in raw meat. In wild animals who consume raw meat, enzymes keep blood vessels clear of fatty deposits by promoting proper breakdown of fats in the digestive tract and liver. When researcher Dr. Maynard Murray dissected more than 3,000 whales that had a 3–6-inch layer of fat around their bodies, he found no signs of circulatory disease.[10] Their diet is raw fish.

In 1926, Dr. William T. Lopp studied primitive Eskimos and found no signs of kidney or vascular diseases.[10] In adult Eskimos (40–60 years old), the average blood pressure reading was 129/76. More civilized Eskimos who settled in the Hudson Bay area, close to trading posts, used cooked food and white-flour products. They gave up their primitive diet—and consequently, their good health. Arteriosclerosis and high blood pressure now occur among these people. The largest factor differentiating primitive and civilized Eskimos is diet.

Absorption, Antigens, and Allergies

Various undesirable substances can be absorbed through the intestinal wall into the bloodstream. At the University of Illinois, feeding compressed yeast to dogs produced positive yeast cultures in the liver, lymph glands, lungs, spleen, and kidneys, proving that whole yeast cells were absorbed.[11] It is well known that undigested proteins, yeast, carbohydrates, and fats can be absorbed into the bloodstream, causing allergies, skin diseases, and other illnesses.[6,30]

Foods that don't get digested properly can cause undesirable reactions. For example, Dr. Oelgoetz showed that undigested protein, fat, and starch molecules are absorbed into the bloodstream, and when the blood enzyme level is below normal, these unassimilated molecules can cause allergies. By giving amylase, protease, and lipase orally to his patients, their blood enzyme level was normalized and the allergies were alleviated.[26]

There are many similarities in the cause and prevention of allergies and candida infection. Basically, the symptoms of both maladies are due to the body's attempt to resist the microorganisms, toxins, or other substances that tend to damage tissues and organs—that is, basic immune responses.

A major part of the immune system is several types of white blood cells, such as lymphocytes (including T-cells and B-cells), macrophages, T-cells, B-cells, and neutrophils. They differ slightly in their duties. T-lymphocytes, for example, become sensitized to specific antigens (substances that cause an immune response) and attack them whenever they're found in the body. B-lymphocytes produce antibodies, which are specific molecules that attach to specific antigens to aid in their destruction.

White blood cells help to destroy antigens and other toxins by engulfing them and digesting or partially destroying them, making it easier for the body to eliminate them. In most cases, they do this by secreting enzymes that break down the antigens. Previously mentioned experiments by Dr. Willstatter proved as far back as 1933 that white blood cells contain eight different types of amylase, protease, and lipase. He states, "White blood cells provide transportation for enzymes throughout the body."[40]

Antigens, bacteria, yeast, and other toxins often enter the body through the digestive tract, often in food substances, and then multiply prolifically if the immune system is not strong and healthy enough to destroy them. Allergens (substances that cause an allergic response) can also enter the body through the air we breathe. It is important to note that antigens, bacteria, viruses, and yeasts are proteins. Often, bacteria secrete protein-containing toxins that also allergies and immune responses.

At this point, you should be able to see that the body needs a tremendous supply of protein-digestive enzymes to counteract and eliminate the constant bombardment of these proteins. Enzymatic protein digestion occurs not only in the digestive tract but in the bloodstream, where undigested proteins are often found if food digestion was not properly accomplished.

Other allergens can attach themselves to these proteins in the bloodstream, forming antigen complexes that can be deposited in capillary walls, where they secrete substances that cause inflammation. This results in swelling, sneezing, hay fever, hives, asthma, and so forth. For the body to get rid of the allergen, it must be separated from the protein molecule by a protein-digestive enzyme and eliminated via the lymphatic system. This is why it is so important to keep the lymphatic system clean.

The toxic effects of undigested proteins, bacteria, and yeast entering the bloodstream via the intestinal wall cannot be stressed strongly enough. Their quick proliferation often leaves the body with numerous symptoms.

Dealing with Candida Infection

The yeast *Candida albicans* lives naturally in the intestinal tract and other areas of animals and humans. It can take over the whole body if the immune system is weakened, as in advanced cases of AIDS. Candida (and other yeasts/fungi) can change form in the body, either entering the circulation or developing a root structure that penetrates the intestinal wall, creating a large enough opening for other micro-organisms and antigens (such as undigested protein) to enter.

These antigens and other invading substances are a major cause of allergies, anxiety, fatigue, digestive disturbances, vaginitis, cystitis, menstrual problems, and migraine. That is the reason for the similar approach in treating candida and allergies: it is important to realize that yeasts are protein bodies and can be digested by enzymes if the body has a proper supply. Yeast and many other proteinaceous antigens can be eliminated by administering supplemental enzymes. These supplements nourish white blood cells, causing a direct improvement of immune system function.

As mentioned, some allergens are not protein themselves but are combined with protein molecules. Undigested proteins, to which yeast and other allergens attach themselves in the circulation, often enter by way of the digestive tract. One way to prevent this is to take plant-derived proteolytic enzymes with meals to aid in their digestion. An effective approach to existing candida infection, allergies, or any other systemic problem is to take plant enzymes between meals and thereby help to increase enzyme activity throughout the body, thus reestablishing these levels in both the digestive tract and bloodstream.

Again, simply eating larger amounts of raw foods, taking supplemental enzymes, and taking the herb echinacea can help to alleviate problems of this type. You can also use *Lactobacillus acidophilus* to check the spread of yeast in the intestines and nourish the immune system.

Certain toxins, viruses, bacteria, parasites, and fungi, and other antigens cause inflammatory reactions. When immune complexes (antigens and antibodies combined) overaccum-ulate in the bloodstream, they can be deposited in tissues. Inflammation begins, and leads to allergy or even tissue destruction. This process can affect the intestinal tract, causing Crohn's disease or ulcerative colitis. The list of consequences is endless. Immune complexes can be reduced by using hydrolytic (bond-splitting) proteolytic enzymes. This is very effective to reduce the inflammation of allergic reactions.

Dr. Howell explains that food allergies result when protease, amylase, and lipase in the blood fall below a certain level, allowing undigested food substances to accumulate in the blood.[10] Taking a complete enzyme formula between meals restores the proper blood enzyme level. Undigested food particles can then be eliminated, and the food allergies can be overcome. Any food can cause an allergy. The most common are milk, eggs, shellfish, wheat, soy, peanuts, and other kinds of fish. I've also seen coffee allergies. It's up to our immune system to protect us. The immune system produces antibodies such as the immunoglobulin IgE, "the allergy antibody," in response to allergens. This sets off a chain of events that cause symptoms known as allergic reactions. Any disease can be caused by long-term allergies and inflammation.

Other Invaders

Parasites are an often-overlooked cause of inflammation and allergy. It has been said that 50–70 percent of our population has parasites. Parasites that take up residence in our bloodstream and elsewhere in the body can live off foods, chemicals, and even gases, and have been known to swell up to twice their size from whatever they're living on. They can cause inflammation throughout our bodies. Parasite eggs are virtually everywhere. One study showed 50 percent of all vegetables carry parasites![32] This is one of the reasons why it is so important to wash all produce very thoroughly.

Allergy researcher Dr. Alan Hunter showed that parasites are heat-sensitive, meaning that a high body temperature can control or eliminate them. A low body temperature, such as in low-thyroid conditions, enhances their activity.[12] If you do have allergies, get tested for parasites and check your temperature throughout the day. One degree makes a big difference in the body.

Recommendations for Health

We live such unnatural lifestyles; we create disease from within. Why do I eat a tomato and don't get an allergic reaction, but the person next to me does? The problem is somewhere within our individual selves, or we'd all be allergic to the same things. If you're genetically prone to inflammation, allergy, or disease, adjust your foods and lifestyle appropriately. You're unique; find out what is right for you. It takes guts to be healthy!

We're different at many levels, but we can all do some basic things to keep ourselves balanced. First, clean up. There are all sorts of cleansing diets and herbs. (See *Natural Healing with Herbs* and *Your Body Speaks—Your Body Heals* for suggestions to start with.) We should all do cleansing diets once in a while. Eat—or drink!—fresh, raw fruits and vegetables daily, as 40–60 percent of your diet.

Two supplements I strongly suggest for daily, long-term use are digestive enzymes and probiotics. If inflammation is a problem, find a good health practitioner and deal with it. If it's in a specific body part, use appropriate herbs and diet. The herb echinacea, a lymphatic cleanser, is excellent in combination with enzymes, because it stimulates the production of white blood cells. It's used to treat inflammation, lymphatic swelling, allergy, and infection. Use proteolytic enzymes between meals to help eliminate infections and inflammation.

Give up bad habits. Stay away from substances that cause inflammation, such as coffee, cigarettes, high-acid foods—and by all means, stay hydrated! A lot of us are dehydrated, which is a major contributor to inflammation.

Recommendations for a General Anti-Inflammatory Program

- using digestive enzymes with meals
- using proteolytic enzymes between meals
- using Juice Plus+® products (especially Vineyard Blend®)
- keeping hydrated
- increase vegetables and minimizing fruit
- using buffered vitamin C
- using lipoic acid
- using methylsulfonylmethane (MSM)
- monitoring your salivary and urinary pH (see below)

You can also add herbs and other specific supplements for particular needs. Find a good health practitioner to help with proper dosages. (Use the system detailed in *ProMetabolics: Your Personal Guide to Transformational Health and Healing* to monitor your pH, your body's response to diet and supplements, your hormonal balance, and more.)

WHO NEEDS ENZYMES

"Do I need more enzymes?" This is a question that only the individual can answer, according to his or her own knowledge and understanding, and with the consideration of certain facts. For example, there's the fact that aging correlates with a decreasing enzyme reserve in the body; therefore, doing all you can to maintain and increase enzyme levels would be beneficial toward increased tissue and organ longevity. There's also the fact that during all acute and chronic illnesses, enzymes are used up more rapidly than usual, and therefore increasing enzyme intake would be beneficial if you are sick or recovering. People with health problems ranging from stress, hypoglycemia, and obesity to endocrine deficiencies, anorexia nervosa, and many others could all benefit from more enzymes.

Enzymes Enhance Other Supplementation

The utilization of vitamins depends upon enzymes, and enzymes often depend on vitamins. Under clinical observation, it has been shown that when vitamins and minerals are combined in capsules with enzymes, smaller amounts of vitamins and minerals are needed. I saw this phenomenon in a patient of mine who needed 70 milligrams of supplemental zinc daily to overcome a severe depletion. When zinc was combined with certain enzymes, this patient needed only 3 micrograms daily—a very drastic reduction in supplementation.

We're all interested in saving money, and it's possible to reduce our intake of vitamin and mineral supplements while maintaining our daily requirements. Many clinicians have learned that a patient is more likely to follow a health regimen if it can be made as easy and as practical as possible.

Detoxification

Numerous methods are used to detoxify the body: fasting, purging, vegetarian or macrobiotic diets, "the grape cure," and many others. All of these have been successful for some people on their own. But none of these regimes will work all the time. What can be done to improve all these cleansing methods? Enzymes can be used not only to maintain health, but also during detoxification programs and in medical and nonmedical approaches to healing. They can be a support system for the entire body and all health-promotion processes.

Any time cooked food is eaten, it must be digested by enzymes. Then, leftover wastes and any toxins from the food are broken down by scavenger enzymes of the immune system. The body draws enzymes from all of its tissue resources for these jobs. Heavy starches (such as bread), animal proteins, and fried foods are more difficult to break down, requiring more enzymes. This is why a vegetarian diet is often used for cleansing. Many are raw-food diets, which contribute enzymes to the enzyme-stomach as well as the rest of the body. But even cooked vegetables and grains, which use some of the body's enzymes, are easier to digest than more concentrated foods.

The energy required to break down food, extract the nutrients, and eliminate waste products while on a cleansing diet—especially if raw juices and predigested foods are used—is far less than the energy required to digest the everyday, traditional, nearly enzyme-free cooked diet. I've seen tremendous recoveries using predigested-food diets of raw sprouts, fresh-squeezed juices, and soaked seeds and nuts (soaked 4–8 hours minimum) that are blended before being eaten.

As previously described, two major changes take place in predigestion: the food is broken into simpler components—proteins into amino acids, starches into simpler sugars, and fats into fatty acids; and the food's enzyme content increases, sometimes tenfold. Predigested foods donate enzymes, relieve the body of the burden of breaking down concentrated foods, and conserve energy and enzymes for other metabolic functions, such as cleansing.

Detoxification is intended to clean the bloodstream and balance the endocrine glands so they work in harmony instead of being overstimulated and exhausted. This purifies the organs and tissues and takes stress off the entire body. Within the bloodstream and body tissues, enzymes act as scavengers, breaking down cholesterol and other fatty deposits and assisting in the overall detoxification process.

Enzymes for "Healing Crisis" Recovery and Bowel Cleansing

I've mentioned that enzymes, as a part of the immune system, break down toxins and various accumulations in our bodies. When there is a shortage of lipase in the blood, for instance, cholesterol can accumulate. It seems logical, then, that any enzyme-increasing diet would aid in purification, especially as enzymes can be reabsorbed and reused by the body.

Many authors have written about the "healing crisis" (it's covered thoroughly in *Your Body Speaks—Your Body Heals*). A healing crisis occurs when the system is overloaded with toxins and the body works to eliminate them through the skin, bowels, sinuses, kidneys, and lungs, producing such symptoms as rashes, congestion, constipation, diarrhea, and urinary tract problems. All of these are symptoms of body cleansing. Tissues releasing poisons that have been stored for years may even contain drugs ingested long ago.

During these crises, enzymes are busy breaking down wastes so the body can rid itself of them. It would seem that adding enzymes during a healing crisis could only be beneficial and aid in cleansing, and this has proven to be true. (To research this topic, read Dr. Edward Howell's *Food Enzymes for Health and Longevity* and *Enzyme Nutrition: The Food Enzyme Concept.*[10,11])

Sometimes detoxification actually weakens the person, even though a good cleansing diet has been prescribed. If patients have a weak constitution or a chronic disease, or are easily discouraged, they tend to go back to their old diet as soon as the first healing crisis is experienced. They think the cleansing diet isn't worth it because it makes them feel worse, even if only temporarily. When poisons eliminated from the tissues enter the bloodstream, the endocrine glands secrete hormones, which in turn affect the eliminative organs, resulting in a feeling of stimulation. When the glands become overworked and exhausted, there will be a feeling of exhaustion, and recovery time will be necessary. These people really need enzyme support.

Using supplemental enzymes and predigested foods will take much of the stress from these patients' systems. They also need a good learning process in relation to healthful eating habits, fasting, and the proper use of colonics and enemas as adjuncts to healing. Bowel cleansing is one of the first measures considered by natural healing practitioners.

The bowel is the "sewage system" of the body, and it too must be cleaned out. It has been estimated that 80 percent of all diseases start in the large bowel. What generally happens is that undigested food putrefies in the colon, producing by-products that are absorbed through the intestinal wall into the bloodstream and deposited in the joints and other tissues. Enzymes can help with this, as Dr. Selle has shown that adding enzymes to the diet reduces fecal bulk, speeds transit time, and can reduce potentially stinky nitrogen compounds (found in high-protein foods) 30–60 percent.[11]

Infants and Children

Many diseases in early stages of development are promoted by the ingestion of foods lacking the vitamins, minerals, and enzymes needed daily by the body. Manufacturing procedures, depleted soils, and cooking create undernutrition. I have emphasized counteracting the enzyme deficiency that often occurs with age, but young people need enzymes too.

Complete breast-feeding of infants is very important. Mother's milk has all the nutrients needed for the growth of a child, along with a large amount of live enzymes, which a baby thrives upon. Milk formulas lack enzymes, and artificial formulas can even be toxic, promoting infections, mucus conditions, fevers, diarrhea, colic, and allergies.

Over a period of years at a clinic operated by the Infant Welfare Society of Chicago, the health and development of 20,061 infants was closely monitored for the first 9 months of their lives. Of the total, 48.5 percent were wholly breast-fed, 43 percent partially breast-fed, and 8.5 percent wholly artificially fed. Table 2 shows the mortality rates of these groups:

	# Infants	# Deaths	% Mortality
Wholly breast-fed	9,749	15	0.5
Partially breast-fed	8,605	59	0.7
Artificially fed	1,707	144	8.4

Table 2

Note that the mortality rate for the artificially fed infants was *56 times greater* than among the breast-fed. Four of the 9,749 breast-fed infants died of respiratory infections, compared to 82 of the 1,707 artificially fed infants.[7]

In the United States, one deformed child is born every 5 minutes, which is the equivalent of one in every ten families. That's 250,000 deformed infants yearly, 75 percent of whom have mental defects. When considering an infant's health, a major factor is the mother's health. In *Food Is Your Best Medicine*, Dr. Henry G. Bieler states, "Unless the mother is detoxified before conceiving, the baby comes into the world...full of toxins from the mother's blood and an intestine full of meconium (black bile). The baby is, in fact, so toxic that even with the best care it usually takes three years to eliminate his or her inherited birth poisons."[2]

Another factor is that a baby brought into the world with a weak constitution and a poison-laden bloodstream is then expected to exist on a diet of concentrated, enzyme-free foods. Heavy starches and mucus-inducing foods (such as dairy products, grains, and sugar) bring on respiratory disorders, asthma, pneumonia, measles, and runny noses. Eating excessively fatty food brings on high-cholesterol problems, acne, and boils.

Doctors have recently begun to examine school children for high cholesterol and triglycerides. The foods most school children consume lack the three major enzymes—lipase, protease, and amylase—that help break down foods in the digestive tract. This results in the absorption of large protein and fat molecules, which lay the foundation for allergies, obesity, constipation, and fatigue.

Two of the major problems now faced by school systems are hyperactivity and absenteeism. It is very difficult for children to learn when they cannot concentrate. The relationship between the mind and what the body eats is of paramount importance. Learning disabilities are often caused by nutrient deficiencies, and the majority of these deficiencies are caused by foods that lack enzymes—too much cooked food, junk food, processed food, and the like. The child's body becomes toxic and the nerves become irritated.

Two children out of every 100 have a neurological disorder observable by medical examination. But what about the child who doesn't exhibit a recognized disorder but suffers from an overstimulated nervous system caused by soft drinks, caffeine in chocolate bars, sugar, or other stimulants? Haven't you ever experienced the jitters when you've had too much coffee or sugar? A child's body is much more sensitive than an adult's; in some cases, even the mere use of salt can cause hyperactivity, dehydration, and allergies.

Children who maintain high enzyme levels maintain high energy levels. Consider the many ways growing children and young adults lose enzymes. During all fevers and infections, the immune system uses large amounts of enzymes to protect the body and eliminate toxins and bacteria. In fact, as previously stated, any time the temperature of the body is raised, enzymes are used up—during healthy exercise as well as during fever. More calories are burned during exercise, and their natural oxidation is initiated by enzymes.

Overfeeding, especially with cooked, devitalized food, causes a child's digestive organs to secrete large amounts of enzymes daily. Over time, this can exhaust the enzyme-producing organs and deplete the immune system, putting a strain on every tissue throughout the body. This child will tend to act exhausted, compared to peers, because his or her energy is being used for digesting foods and coping with the large amounts of waste left over from an unnaturally large food supply. The body is then required to store large amounts of fat, which puts an additional strain on the heart, kidneys, and lungs.

It should be clear that we use up our enzymes in many different ways. The proper thing to do is to feed your child and yourself only when you are hungry. This will conserve enzymes. You and your child should eat most of your food raw and add enzyme supplements to enhance digestion. Consider occasional, short fasts. During fasts, enzymes can focus on cleaning up undigested materials in the blood and purifying the whole body. Then, resume a good, healthy diet; cut out the junk food, and increase fresh fruit and vegetables.

Enzymes and Nutrition for Athletes and Exercisers

What about the athlete, who may be taking vitamins, minerals, and concentrated foods—what makes all of these elements work? Enzymes. Athletes can benefit by taking enzyme supplements, because any time the body temperature is raised, as during exercise, enzymes are used up more rapidly than normal. Carbohydrates are burned more rapidly, and more nutrients are needed for fuel. For an athlete who eats mostly cooked food, this is like burning the candle at both ends. Enzymes are used up rapidly, and little is brought in to replenish the supply.

One of an athlete's main concerns should be what type of food is needed to maintain a healthy body and replace nutrients lost during exercise or competition. Enzymes, carbohydrates, proteins, fats, vitamins, and minerals are the fuels the body needs to function properly. When you exercise, most of these substances are used up rapidly and need replacement.

When I ask people if they feel that their diet is correct in relation to the amount of activity they are involved in, their answer is frequently, "Yes, I get plenty of foods high in B vitamins, carbohydrates, proteins, and fats." I've found that these individuals also monitor the nutritional values of foods and calculate their personal needs.

Unfortunately, eating the proper amounts of food and nutrients is only half the battle. Another main concern of an athlete is absorbing and utilizing the food ingested. Food often lacks the proper enzymes—and without enzymes, it cannot be digested completely and the body cannot use its nutrients appropriately. This can result in bloating, fatigue, and stiffness. Arteries harden and undigested fats thicken the blood, reducing the proper utilization of oxygen and cholesterol. The consequences of a lack of enzymes are innumerable; the main point is that enzymes can be a missing link in good nutrition.

A person who exercises regularly is concerned about getting and staying in shape. Strength and endurance are the goals of such individuals. How, then, can anyone achieve endurance if his or her cells are not getting the proper nutrients? Nutrients may be present in foods you eat, but the workforce of the body is enzymes. Most vitamins, for instance, are called coenzymes because they must combine with enzymes before the body can use them.

Over-nutrition and under-absorption result in a low-energy system. People often believe that they don't recover from exercise readily enough because they either overdid it or didn't do enough. The problem may actually be that the engine is congested with unusable fuel.

The more enzymes you take in through eating a good quantity of raw foods and supplementing your diet with enzymes, the more energy you'll have. It's been said that half the body's energy is spent digesting food. If exogenous enzymes (enzymes taken in through food or supplementation) are added to the diet daily, more nutrients will be available and less food will be needed, reducing digestive stress and waste elimination. With this kind of energy conservation, the athlete will be able to work out more often and with greater intensity, and will require less recovery time.

Whenever exercise or sports participation is considered, you must be healthy to carry out the program effectively. You must add to your enzyme reserve, not deplete it. It's great to enjoy sports and other related activities, but it will be a short-lived experience if your metabolic enzyme reserves are not maintained and you fail to supplement the daily losses to your system.

Whether you're an athlete or an exerciser, this information is of paramount importance. If you do not pay close attention to your nutrition, exercise can cause rapid aging rather than help to keep you young and vital. Exercise is a breaking-down and building-up process, and muscle micro-tears and the like from exercise are good—if the body's circulation and nutrition support replacement of the damaged tissue with new, elastic tissue.

When it comes to inflammation, the immune system acts the same during exercise as during disease. It is very dependent on enzymes in regard to inflammation and protection from damage. Hormone-like cytokines are involved in cell-to-cell communication, such as immune system interactions. A change in certain cytokine levels is of specific interest, as it allows us to recognize immune system imbalances.

A balance between the two cytokine categories, Th1 and Th2, indicates optimal health. Th1 cytokines produce inflammation in response to exercise, bacterial, viral, and fungal responses. This is a normal, healthy response. But uncontrolled, this response can perpetuate tissue-damaging immune reactions. During acute inflammation, Th2 cytokines are the anti-inflammatory responders and counteract Th1. Another good thing. Th2 is found to be high during asthma, eczema, allergic imbalances, and other inflammations.

Removal of Th1 cytokines to downgrade inflammation is mediated by proteolytic enzymes. These enzymes combine with a carbohydrate-protein compound (glycoprotein), and this new complex has the capacity to bind with Th1 and other cytokines, facilitating their removal. This enzyme complex also binds with proteins damaged by oxidative stress. During exercise, proteins in muscle fibers are broken down, free radicals are produced, and oxidative stress is created. To counter this damage, I often suggest taking extra proteolytic enzymes between meals, eating plenty of fruits and vegetables, and taking extra antioxidants. (Juice Plus+®, especially the Vineyard Blend®, is excellent for this purpose. See *Your Body Speaks — Your Body Heals.*)

Back to cytokines. Once they're back in balance, regeneration takes place. The importance of systemic enzymes cannot be denied during this process. The oral administration of exogenous proteolytic enzymes such as trypsin, chymotrypsin, and the plant enzymes bromelain and papain will help keep us young. (The National Enzyme Company in Forsyth, MO, offers wonderful enzymes; see www.nationalenzyme.com.)

Joint health is improved tremendously by using enzyme support. Research has shown enzymes to be as effective as some nonsteroidal anti-inflammatory drugs (NSAIDS), especially for sports injuries and their prevention, hip and knee injuries, and preserving joint cartilage damage.[1,8] Wonder why there are so many hip and knee replacements as we get older? When we exercise and train, we're literally tearing down our joints, sweating out minerals, and creating oxidative stress (free radical damage). In other words, we age!

Here again are my recommendations for a General Anti-Inflammatory Program.

Recommendations for a General Anti-Inflammatory Program

- using digestive enzymes with meals
- using proteolytic enzymes between meals
- using Juice Plus+® products (especially Vineyard Blend®)
- keeping hydrated
- increase vegetables and minimizing fruit
- using buffered vitamin C
- using lipoic acid
- using methylsulfonylmethane (MSM)
- monitoring your salivary and urinary pH (see below)

You can also add herbs and other specific supplements for particular needs. Find a good health practitioner to help with proper dosages. (Use the system detailed in *ProMetabolics: Your Personal Guide to Transformational Health and Healing* to monitor your pH, your body's response to diet and supplements, your hormonal balance, and more.)

JUICING AND JUICE PLUS+®

Raw foods put you back in touch with food's real taste, real texture, and whole fiber. Eating raw foods allows you to keep a good balance of enzymes in your system as well. When you combine a diet higher in raw foods with the use of juicing, you get the added advantage of concentrated vitamins and minerals in a readily bioavailable form.

Raw Juice

Starting in the 1940s and continuing well into the 50s and 60s, naturopathic physician Dr. Norman Walker, "the guru of juicing," helped thousands of people regain their health through the use of juice.[37] Another physician of the time, Dr. Max Gerson, also emphasized juice in treatment for chronic illnesses. He believed that administering uncooked food in the form of "live" juice was the fastest way to help rejuvenate the body of an ill person, and he had his patients drink 8–10 ounces of fresh-made carrot and apple juice every 2 hours.[35]

Drinking fresh fruit and vegetable juices daily as a means of supplying much-needed vitamins, minerals, and enzymes was reemphasized in the 1990s by "the juiceman," Jay Kordich, who saved his own life through dietary changes, particularly juicing. His example and writings encouraged many to take up the practice of consuming juice—as much as 1–3 quarts a day.[19]

Juices put little stress on the digestive tract, because they are easy to absorb and their nutrients are sent into the bloodstream within minutes. Contrast this to the hours it takes to digest a solid meal, and to the small amounts of nutrients available to the body even after several hours of digestion. In addition, most of our foods are already cooked, which destroys 40–60 percent of the amino acids, a large percentage of the minerals, and all the enzymes if cooked at a temperature higher than 120°F. Over the years, we have been feeding ourselves overcooked, deficient food, most likely grown in poor-quality soil. But because juicing uses fresh, uncooked food, these deficiencies are avoided.

Juice can make a remarkable difference for people who are sick. Suddenly, the body is getting fed with easy-to-digest liquid, food/liquid nutrients, and enzymes. That can be a tremendous boost to the immune system, as well as to overall health. Using juice is such a safe and effective way to rebalance the body, no matter what its condition. Juices cleanse the system, rebuild it, and balance it.

The use of juice between meals is one of the most effective ways to cut down on cravings for unhealthy or unnecessary foods. Eating several big meals a day makes us feel dull and diminished. Freeing up the energy used for digestion provides a greater storehouse of healing potential and creative and intellectual activity. We start to feel nourished by the juice in a way we haven't experienced before. Soon, we are also choosing to eat in a way that supports this new form of nourishment.

Juice itself is not a therapy but a foundation for other therapies. Some people can't take heavy supplements or drugs; others can't radically change their eating habits; but almost everybody can start drinking juice.

Juice Recommendations

Fruit juices are "the cleansers" and vegetable juices are "the essential toners and builders." In general, I recommend drinking fruit juice in the morning and vegetable juice in the afternoon and evening. Additionally, I support the use of juices to deal with imbalances in particular bodily systems.

By combining the Western approach to nutrition (in terms of eating, digestion, and the distribution of the nutrients through the glands) with the Eastern or Chinese approach (in terms of energy), I have developed an advanced methodology to determine exactly what foods and juices are good for what parts of the body and what health conditions. (For full details, see *Your Body Speaks—Your Body Heals.*)

A Juicing Alternative

People often start juicing with great enthusiasm but then lose heart and fail to keep up the daily program, because they don't want to take the time or energy to prepare produce for juicing, or their schedules make it difficult to have fresh juices every day, or they travel frequently and easily get out of the juicing habit. Other people are put off from even trying a juicing program by the expense of a high-quality juicer and fresh produce in large quantities. The commitment to better health though food is one that many are unable or unwilling to make.

But I have good news for health-conscious people who need a convenient way to have juice when they work or travel, or who want the health benefits of juicing without the labor. I had long theorized that a powdered juice with the fiber added back to it and enzymes added as well would be a superb addition or alternative to juicing, and some excellent products are now on the market. Furthermore, it is possible to concentrate several types of juice into one capsule or 1 teaspoon of powder, thus providing the nutrients of four to six different vegetables or fruits at once. This can be particularly advantageous for those who are using juice combinations to support specific bodily systems.

For enhancing a child's diet—especially with a child reluctant to eat vegetables and fruits—powdered juices can be the answer to a prayer. Imagine giving your children the benefits of kale, parsley, cabbage, broccoli, and apple, all in a convenient, palatable, powdered form. Although I encourage parents to change their own diets and model eating fresh, raw foods for their children, I know this is difficult for some, impossible for others. So a good powdered juice is the next best thing.

But be forewarned that not all powdered-juice products meet high standards of quality. Some companies simply freeze-dry a concentrated juice, in which the nutrients were already destroyed by cooking/heating. This, in my estimation, is a seriously deficient product. The products I recommend are processed in a way that preserves the original nutrients, and adds fiber and enzymes too.

The Birth of Juice Plus+®

Before I tell you about the research behind Juice Plus+®, I'd like to tell you the personal story that led to the development of this whole-food product. When we're experiencing a trauma or other significant event, we don't always fully understand it until it has passed, and then we realize that it has changed our lives for the better. Living a life is a lesson itself and is always teaching us something; we just have to learn how to interpret the direction it is taking us. Even a chronic illness is pointing us in a specific direction, as I learned when my father got sick.

It was 1980 and I was on a lecture tour, teaching herbal seminars in Denver, CO. During a break, I received a phone call from my father. He told me his spleen had swollen to the size of a football. It was so large he was using one of his Marine Corp belts to hold it up and it was so painful that he could hardly move. My mother made an appointment for him at a nearby hospital, where the doctors could not believe how large his spleen had grown—and it was still growing.

At the end of the day, my dad called me again and said he was diagnosed with lymphoma, cancer of the lymphatic system. I was so stunned I couldn't even reply. I just held the phone, praying that I didn't really hear what he had said. My throat closed up, so tight I could hardly breathe. He felt my shock and distress and told me everything was going to be okay. Being a naturopath and teaching people for years how to live by the laws of nature, I had to ask myself, why did this have to happen? (Don't we all wonder why, when something so traumatic happens to us?)

I told my dad I'd be home in four days as soon as my tour was over. By the time I got there, his doctors had already removed his spleen and started chemotherapy. I was floored, totally irate. No questions had been asked—they just did the surgery and started pumping him full of drugs.

After three weeks, my father had lost 40 pounds and nothing was working. The chemotherapy had failed and there was nothing more they could do. His doctor called our family together and told us my dad had no more than three weeks to live. After breaking the news to my dad, I asked if he'd like to try natural therapy at my clinic in Tucson, AZ, where I would take care of him. He said, "I would have come to you before this, but I didn't want you to be responsible if anything bad would have happened to me." I picked him up and carried him out of the hospital without even checking him out.

By the time we got to Tucson, he weighed 136 pounds, and his cancer was traveling so fast through his body that he couldn't eat or drink. How do you nourish somebody who can't eat or drink? I started massaging him every day with olive oil so his body would absorb the fat through his skin. He could only sip water, so I devised a plan to get more nutrients in through another route. I built a slant-board for him to lie on, made fresh green juice with kale, parsley, and some additional liquid chlorophyll, and used an enema bag to feed him through the bowel with this juice daily.

As he got stronger, he was able to drink vegetable juices by mouth. Fruit juices, however, made him feel ill because of their sugar. You don't want to feed cancer cells sugar, because they thrive on it; plus, it acidifies the body, putting an even greater strain on a sick person's system.

I wanted to find a way to get more concentrated nutrition into his body to increase his strength and boost his healing, and it occurred to me that if I could juice the vegetables and dry the juice, the powder would be more concentrated than the juice itself. I set up some small dryers in my office and found that it would take hours to dry the juice, but it worked. I'd give him tablespoons of vegetable juice powder stirred into small amounts of water daily. To my amazement—keep in mind, at that time we knew nothing about phytochemicals—in two months he put on 30 pounds. There was no meat or carbohydrates other than tablespoons of dried vegetable juice in his diet. I wondered, how could someone put on so much weight without eating?

He then got to the point where he could also drink fruit juice powder without feeling ill, so he'd have fruit juice powder in the morning and vegetable juice powder the rest of the day. I gave him very little fruit juice powder, though, as I noticed that if I gave him too much, his urine's pH would turn acidic. I also added proteolytic enzymes and some herbs to the regime. I was constantly changing the dosages of his supplements according to his pH, using the monitoring system in my book, *ProMetabolics*.

The results were astonishing. Within three months of my taking over his treatment, my father got out of bed and remodeled my kitchen. He had been a carpenter his whole life and loved working with wood. Continuing on a nutritional program of eating large amounts of vegetables, dried juice powders, and soaked and sprouted seeds and nuts, he went back to work within six months and worked as a carpenter for another six years. It's my opinion that he'd still be alive today if his doctors had not removed his spleen and given him such high doses of drugs during his hospitalization.

From my father's recovery, I realized the hidden healing power of whole foods, so I began studying all fruits and vegetables known to man, and I learned that some were much more nutrient-dense than others. Ironically, the ones most concentrated in nutrients were the ones most people didn't eat at all, or always cooked before eating: parsley, beets, cabbage, and broccoli, to name a few.

Experimenting over several months, I created one concentrated juice-powder formula with fruits and another with vegetables—the most nutrient-dense fruits and vegetables on the planet. Soon my clinic looked more like a produce-drying facility, and everyone who came to me, regardless of the problem, was given a bag of each powder. The healings that I observed were no less than miraculous; I knew I was on to something big when my patients were getting well so fast.

The formulas I used in my clinical practice are now the most wonderful line of fruit and vegetable concentrates, called Juice Plus+®. I designed and patented these products, and NSA, Inc. in Memphis, TN, manufactured, distributed, and promoted them. Benefiting thousands of people in over 30 countries, Juice Plus+® is the most researched nutra-ceutical in the world today. (For detailed information, see www.JuicePlus.com.)

Just before my father died, he was so concerned about my professional reputation that he said, "If I die, will people still believe in you? Will they still buy your books?" I said, "Dad, what we accomplished together, this idea of concentrated fruits and vegetables, someday will be known all over the world." And that's exactly what happened. My father's recovery gave birth to the most wonderful product line of fruit and vegetable concentrates, Juice Plus+®.

My father taught me pride and honor. He would tell me that a man's word is all he has. In over 50 years of being a carpenter, he never once had a written contract with anyone—only an agreement of a smile, honor, and love. He will always own a piece of my heart. I know he is always with me; he's my strength and motivation.

The Research Behind Juice Plus+®

I'd like to give special thanks and appreciation to NSA's corporate family and distributors for believing in me and the Juice Plus+® concept, especially President Jay Martin and Vice President John Blair, who are totally responsible for the marketing, research, and distribution of these products. Thanks also go to Jeff Roberti, who introduced me to NSA and was the first person to acknowledge the validity of this concept.

Numerous clinical studies published in peer-reviewed scientific journals have demonstrated the following benefits:

Juice Plus+® delivers key, easily absorbed phytonutrients. Several studies have shown the bioavailability of select nutrients found in Juice Plus+® in a variety of populations. At Tokyo Women's Medical University, Juice Plus+® was shown to increase the bioavailability of various nutrients. (Kawashima A, et al. Four week supplementation with mixed fruit and vegetable juice concentrates increased protective serum antioxidants and folate and decreased plasma homocysteine in Japanese subjects. *Asia Pacific J Clin Nutr* 2007 16:411–21.) The bioavailability of Juice Plus+® was also demonstrated in studies in Europe (Medical University of Vienna and King's College) and Australia (University of Sydney). (Kiefer L, et al. Supplementation with mixed fruit and vegetable juice concentrates increased serum antioxidants and folate in healthy adults. *J Am Coll Nutr* 2004 23:205–11; Leeds AR, et al. Availability of micronutrients from dried, encapsulated fruit and vegetable preparations: a study in healthy volunteers. *J Hum Nutr Dietetics* 2000 13:21–7; Samman S, et al. A mixed fruit and vegetable concentrate increases plasma antioxidant vitamins and folate and lowers plasma homocysteine in men. *J Nutr* 2003 133:2188–93.)

In the United States, the bioavailability of Juice Plus+® has been shown in young adults (University of Florida), middle-aged people (Vanderbilt University School of Medicine), and the elderly (University of Texas Health Science Center). (Nantz MP, et al. Immunity and antioxidant capacity in humans is enhanced by consumption of a dried, encapsulated fruit and vegetable juice concentrate. *J Nutr* 2006 136:2606–10; Houston MC, et al. Juice powder concentrate and systemic blood pressure, progression of coronary artery calcium and antioxidant status in hypertensive subjects: a pilot study. *Evidence-Based Compl Alt Med* 2007 doi:10.1093/ecam/nel108; Wise JA, et al. Changes in plasma carotenoids, alpha-tocopherol, and lipid peroxide levels in response to supplementation with concentrated fruit and vegetable extracts: a pilot study. *Curr Ther Res* 1996 57:445–61.)

Juice Plus+® reduces oxidative stress. Several investigations have reported that Juice Plus+® reduced various markers (signs) of oxidative stress. A study at the University of North Carolina-Greensboro showed that Juice Plus+® Orchard, Garden, and Vineyard Blends® together were effective in reducing a marker of oxidative stress associated with aerobic exercise. (Bloomer RJ, et al. Oxidative stress response to aerobic exercise: comparison of antioxidant supplements. *Med Sci Sports Ex* 2006 38:1098–1105.) Improvements in other markers have been noted in studies of sedentary people in the United States (University of Texas Health Science Center) and England (King's College). (Wise JA, et al. Changes in plasma carotenoids, alpha-tocopherol, and lipid peroxide levels in response to supplementation with concentrated fruit and vegetable extracts: a pilot study. *Curr Ther Res* 1996 57:445–61; Leeds AR, et al. Availability of micronutrients from dried, encapsulated fruit and vegetable preparations: a study in healthy volunteers. *J Human Nutr Dietetics* 2000 13:21–7.)

Juice Plus+® supports the immune system. A healthy immune system protects the body, and good nutrition is critical for a healthy immune system. Clinical studies showed that Juice Plus+® improved several measures of immune function in young adult students at the University of Florida and in elderly people at the University of Arizona. (Nantz MP, et al. Immunity and antioxidant capacity in humans is enhanced by consumption of a dried, encapsulated fruit and vegetable juice concentrate. *J Nutr* 2006 136:2606–10; Inserra PF, et al. Immune function in elderly smokers and nonsmokers improves during supplementation with fruit and vegetable extracts. *Integr Med* 1999 2:3–10.)

Juice Plus+® protects DNA. DNA becomes damaged and fragile when exposed to oxidative stress; a high-quality diet rich in fruits and vegetables (and their antioxidants) helps protect DNA from oxidative damage that can weaken its structural integrity. Studies showed a reduction in DNA damage after taking Juice Plus+® in young adults (University of Florida) and an elderly population (Brigham Young University). (Nantz MP, et al. Immunity and antioxidant capacity in humans is enhanced by consumption of a dried, encapsulated fruit and vegetable juice concentrate. *J Nutr* 2006 136:2606–10; Smith MJ, et al. Supplementation with fruit and vegetable extracts may decrease DNA damage in the peripheral lymphocytes of an elderly population. *Nutr Res* 1999 19:1507–18.)

Juice Plus+® positively affects key cardiovascular indicators. Several investigations have found that Juice Plus+® reduces homocysteine levels. A clinical study at the University of Sydney showed a reduction of homocysteine levels in participants whose levels were already within an acceptable range. (Samman S, et al. A mixed fruit and vegetable concentrate increases plasma antioxidant vitamins and folate and lowers plasma homocysteine in men. *J Nutr* 2003 133:2188–93.) Researchers in Foggia, Italy, found that Juice Plus+® reduced homocysteine levels in participants whose levels had been elevated. (Panunzio MF, et al. Supplementation with fruit and vegetable concentrate decreases plasma homocysteine in a dietary controlled trial. *Nutr Res* 2003 23:1221–8.)

Researchers at the University of Maryland found that participants who consumed Juice Plus+® were better able to maintain elasticity of their arteries, even after a high-fat meal. (Plotnick GD, et al. Effect of supplemental phytonutrients on impairment of the flow-mediated brachial artery vasoactivity after a single high-fat meal. *J Am Coll Cardiol* 2003 41:1744–9.)

Investigators at Vanderbilt University School of Medicine monitored several measures of vascular health in a low-risk population taking Juice Plus+® for two years, and noted modest improvements with no adverse side effects. (Houston MC, et al. Juice powder concentrate and systemic blood pressure, progression of coronary artery calcium and antioxidant status in hypertensive subjects: a pilot study. *Evidence-Based Compl Alt Med* 2007 doi:10.1093/ecam/nel108.)

Examples of Current and Past Juice Plus+® Research Affiliations

Brigham Young University
Georgetown University
King's College, London, England
Medical University of Graz, Austria
Medical University of Vienna, Austria
Tokyo Women's Medical University, Japan
University of Arizona
University of Birmingham, England
University of California, Los Angeles
University of Florida
University of Maryland School of Medicine
University of Milan, Italy
University of Mississippi Medical Center
University of North Carolina-Greensboro
University of South Carolina
University of Sydney, Australia
University of Texas Health Science Center
University of Texas/MD Anderson
University of Würzburg, Germany
Vanderbilt University School of Medicine
Wake Forest University (with NCI-National Institutes of Health)
Yale University-Griffin Hospital Prevention Research Center

ABOUT THE AUTHOR

Dr. Humbart "Smokey" Santillo, N.D., is recognized as a visionary and pioneer in the growing field of Natural Therapeutics. He is the author of eight books—including the bestselling *Food Enzymes: The Missing Link to Radiant Health* and *Natural Healing with Herbs, ProMetabolics: Your Personal Guide to Transformational Health and Healing,* and his latest,— *Your Body Speaks—Your Body Heals,* read by more than 3.5 million people worldwide. A member of the Naturopathic Medical Association, he holds several patents in the field of nutrition and is highly sought after by sports shows and talk shows.

Born and raised in Lockport, New York, Dr. Santillo received a Bachelor of Science degree from Edinboro State Teacher's College in Pennsylvania, attending on football and track scholarships.

He subsequently developed 33 allergies and the early stages of rheumatoid arthritis; three years of suffering through traditional treatments with little or no relief launched his passionate, life-long quest for better health. Seeking answers and alternatives, he earned the degrees of Doctor of Naturopathy, Health Practitioner, and Master Herbalist. With his own health restored, he has since offered counseling and healing to more than 30,000 patients through his practice.

At the 1995 U.S. Track and Field World Masters Games, comprising 6,400 athletes from 74 countries, Dr. Santillo anchored his 4 x 100-meter relay team to a gold medal victory. In the same year he broke two state records in the 100- and 200-meter races at the Empire State Games in New York, and won both the 100- and 200-meter races in the Canadian Nationals. He continues to compete today, taking first place in the 100-meter race at the 2008 New Jersey State Finals, and first place in the 100-meter Masters race at the 2009 Tampa Bay "Beat the Heat."

REFERENCES

1. Akhtar NM, et al. Oral enzyme combination versus diclofenac in the treatment of osteoarthritis of the knee – a double-blind prospective randomized study. *Clinical Rheumatology.* 2004, 23:410–5.
2. Bieler HG. *Food Is Your Best Medicine.* 1965, Random House, New York, NY.
3. Bjorksten J. A common molecular basis for the aging syndrome. *Journal of the American Geriatrics Society.* 1958, 6:740–7.
4. Cannon WB. Recent advances in the knowledge of the movements and innervation of the alimentary canal. *Medical News.* 1905, 86:923–9.
5. Crandall LA. The origin and significance of the blood serum enzymes. *American Journal of Digestive Diseases.* 1935, 2:230–5.
6. Fisher V. Intestinal absorption of viable yeast. *Proceedings of the Society for Experimental Biology and Medicine.* 1930, 28:948–51.
7. Grulee CG, et al. Breast and artificial feeding influence on morbidity and mortality of twenty thousand infants. *Journal of the American Medical Association.* 1934, 103:735–9.
8. Guseinov NI. Wobenzym in therapy of rheumatoid arthritis. *International Journal on Immunorehabilitation.* 2001, 3:73–4.
9. Hennrich N, et al. [Suitability of the plant protease bromelain for substitution therapy in digestive disorders]. [Article in German] *Arzneimittelforschung.* 1965, 15:434–7.
10. Howell E. *Enzyme Nutrition: The Food Enzyme Concept.* 1985, Avery Publishing Group, Wayne, NJ.
11. Howell E. *Food Enzymes for Health and Longevity.* 1980, Omangod Press, Woodstock Valley, CT.

12. Hunter A. Food/chemical allergies: an original discovery. *Townsend Letter for Doctors and Patients*. 2004, 255(Oct.):67–74.

13. Ingle L, et al. A study of longevity, growth, reproduction and heart rate in *Daphnia longispina* as influenced by limitations in quantity of food. *Journal of Experimental Zoology*. 1937, 76:325–52.

14. Ivy AC, et al. On the effectiveness of malt amylase on the gastric digestion of starches. *Journal of Nutrition*. 1936, 12:59–83.

15. Johnson CE, Wies CH. Influence of ligation of pancreatic ducts of dogs upon serum amylase concentration. *Journal of Experimental Medicine*. 1932, 55:505–9.

16. Keohane PP, et al. Influence of protein composition and hydrolysis method on intestinal absorption of protein in man. *Gut*. 1985, 26: 907–13.

17. Kim YS, Brophy EJ. Effect of amino acids on purified rat intestinal brush-border membrane aminooligopeptidase. *Gastroenterology*. 1979, 76:82–7.

18. Kohman EF, et al. Comparative experiments with canned, home cooked, and raw food diets. *Journal of Nutrition*. 1937, 14:9–19.

19. Kordich J. *The Juiceman's Power of Juicing*. 1992, William Morrow, New York, NY.

20. Kouchakoff P. The influence of food cooking on the blood formula of man. 1930, Proceedings: First International Congress of Microbiology, Paris. Institute of Clinical Chemistry, Lausanne, Switzerland.

21. Kulvinskas V. *Survival Into the 21st Century*. 1975, Omangod Press, Wethersfield, CT.

22. Kunze R. Unpublished studies, 1997.

23. Lepkovsky S, Furuta F. Lipase in pancreas and intestinal contents of chickens fed heated and raw soybean diets.

Poultry Science. 1970, 49:192–8.

24. Maseri A. Inflammation, atherosclerosis, and ischemic events—exploring the hidden side of the moon. *New England Journal of Medicine.* 1997, 336:1014–6.

25. McDougall JA, McDougall MA. *The McDougall Plan.* 1983, New Century Publishers, Piscataway, NJ.

26. Oelgoetz AW, et al. The treatment of food allergy and indigestion of pancreatic origin with pancreatic enzymes. *American Journal of Digestive Diseases and Nutrition.* 1935, 2:422.

27. Pottenger FM, Jr. *Pottenger's Cats: A Study in Nutrition.* 1995, Price-Pottenger Nutrition Foundation, Lemon Grove, CA.

28. Pryor WA. *Introduction to Free Radical Chemistry.* 1966, Prentice-Hall, Englewood Cliffs, NJ.

29. Rachmilewitz M. Blood diastase in hepatic and biliary disease. *American Journal of Digestive Diseases.* 1938, 5:184–9.

30. Ratner B, Gruehl HL. Passage of native proteins through the normal gastro-intestinal wall. *Journal of Clinical Investigation.* 1934, 13:517–32.

31. Ridker PM, et al. Inflammation, aspirin, and the risk of cardiovascular disease in apparently healthy men. *New England Journal of Medicine.* 1997, 336:973–9.

32. Rude RA, et al. Survey of fresh vegetables for nematodes, amoebae, and Salmonella. *Journal of the Association of Official Analytical Chemists.* 1984, 67:613–5.

33. Schmerel F. [Ueber die verminderte Diastasewirkung des Harns bei Nierenerkrankungen und beim Diabetes.] *Biochemische Zeitschrift.* 1929, 208:415–27.

34. Selle WA, Moody IW. The effect of enteric-coated pancreatin on fat and protein digestion of depancreatized dogs. *Journal of Nutrition.* 1937, 13:15–28.

35. Straus H. *Dr. Max Gerson: Healing the Hopeless.* 2001, Quarry Books, Kingston, Ontario, Canada.

36. Taylor WH. Studies on gastric proteolysis. I. The proteolytic activity of human gastric juice and pig and calf gastric mucosal extracts below pH 5. *Biochemistry Journal.* 1959, 71:73–83.

37. Walker NW. *Raw Vegetable Juices: What's Missing in Your Body?* 1970, Norwalk Press, Phoenix, AZ.

38. Werbach MR. *Nutritional Influences on Illness: A Sourcebook of Clinical Research.* 1988, Keats Publishing, New Canaan, CT.

39. Willstatter R. Problems of modern enzyme chemistry. *Chemical Reviews.* 1933, 13:501–12.

40. Willstatter R, Rohdewald M. Uber die Amylasen der Leukocyten. II. [Neunte Abhandlung über Enzyme der Leukocyten.] *Zeitschrift fur Physiologische Chemie.* 1933, 221:13–32.

41. Wolf M, Ransberger K. *Enzyme Therapy.* 1977, Regent House, Los Angeles, CA.

INDEX

D

E

H

I

V

W

Y

yeast, 29, 85–88
Your Body Speaks – Your Body Heals (Santillo), 90, 95, 103, 107

Z

zinc, 69
zukemono, 44

ORDER FORM

Name: _____

Address: _____

_____

Phone: _____

Email Address: _____

	Quantity	Price	Total
Power of Enzymes	_____	14.95	_____
Your Body Speaks...	_____	12.95	_____
ProMetabolics	_____	29.95	_____
Natural Healing with Herbs	_____	16.95	_____

(Call for shipping price for your order)

TOTAL _____

Mail: Vartabedian & Associates, P.O. Box 1671, Carlsbad, CA 92018
Phone: 888-796-5229
Fax: 760-804-5996
Online: www.SmokeySantillo.com

Card #: _____   Exp.:_____

✓ one: ❑ MC ❑ VISA ❑ AMEX ❑ Discover   CVV2: _____

Signature: _____

ORDER FORM

Name: _____

Address: _____

_____

Phone: _____

Email Address: _____

	Quantity	Price	Total
Power of Enzymes	_____	14.95	_____
Your Body Speaks...	_____	12.95	_____
ProMetabolics	_____	29.95	_____
Natural Healing with Herbs	_____	16.95	_____

(Call for shipping price for your order)

TOTAL _____

Mail: Vartabedian & Associates, P.O. Box 1671, Carlsbad, CA 92018
Phone: 888-796-5229
Fax: 760-804-5996
Online: www.SmokeySantillo.com

Card #: _____ Exp.:_____

✓ one: ❏ MC ❏ VISA ❏ AMEX ❏ Discover CVV2:_____

Signature: _____